THE
SECRET
OF
RESILIENCE

"It is time to remember your sacred wholeness as a human being—drawing on your innate wisdom for resilience and well-being. Through intimate stories and sacred principles, you will understand that you are a vital part of the Hoop of Life. If you wish to be more resilient and to be the ambassador of your well-being then read *The Secret of Resilience*."

ANITA SANCHEZ, PH.D., AUTHOR OF *THE FOUR SACRED GIFTS*

"This is a book for the times in which we live. *The Secret of Resilience* will surprise you with its simplicity, accessibility, humanity, and beauty. Stephanie presents us with a path forward that feels both possible and necessary. This is a must-read for those who are awake to what is ahead for us."

CLARE DUBOIS, FOUNDER OF TREESISTERS

"Stephanie Mines's numinous and lyrical memoir gorgeously embodies healing in Interbeing. Its profound truths shift our understanding of what it means to be human, especially as we relate to birth, Gaia, and cosmos. It will unwind the fields of trauma, bodywork, acupuncture, embryology, and all of medicine."

STELLA OSOROJOS EISENSTEIN, DAOM, IMT

"It is hard work weaving poetry into the gritty work of healing trauma, but Mines has managed to produce a book that is both medicinal *and* mystical."

SOPHIE STRAND, AUTHOR OF *THE FLOWERING WAND*
AND *THE MADONNA SECRET*

"*The Secret of Resilience* brings decades of academic and personal insight into focus from an embryological and neurodevelopmental standpoint. As Mines states, we have a birthright of resilience. This book is sure to be of enormous help to many people wading out of the muck of trauma into this inheritance."

TRISTA HENDREN, PUBLISHER OF GIRL GOD BOOKS

"This book is an 'allegiance to the earth' and an invitation to reunite with our birthright."

CHERYL PALLANT, PH.D., AUTHOR OF *ECOSOMATICS*

"This book appears at the precise time that it is needed for planetary evolution. Mines has dedicated her life to a brilliant exploration of embryology. In that exploration, she has found the secret to resilience that is the key to meeting these chaotic and heartbreaking times. Her personal and professional message directs us to the rediscovery of our innate brilliance. This is a must-read for anyone who inhabits a body and is curious about why they are here now."

DR. CLARE WILLOCKS, OB-GYN, FOUNDER OF
BRIDGING THE HEALTHCARE GAP

"It is so rare and precious to find a teacher who prefers not to *tell* you things, so much as *sing* you into a new realm of knowledge and vision. Stephanie Mines is a dancer: she dances from the most touchingly and disarmingly personal to the grandest visions for humanity's potential future. She calls us fearlessly to a homecoming, a necessary return to our ecstatic inner core: our limitless source of vitality and renewal. I've learned so much from this tender and compassionate book. It's exactly the book humanity needs today."

ROBIN GRILLE, PSYCHOLOGIST AND AUTHOR OF
PARENTING FOR A PEACEFUL WORLD AND
INNER CHILD JOURNEYS

THE
SECRET
OF
RESILIENCE

HEALING PERSONAL
AND PLANETARY TRAUMA
THROUGH MORPHOGENESIS

A Sacred Planet Book

STEPHANIE MINES, PH.D.

Healing Arts Press
Rochester, Vermont

Healing Arts Press
One Park Street
Rochester, Vermont 05767
www.HealingArtsPress.com

Healing Arts Press is a division of Inner Traditions International

Sacred Planet Books are curated by Richard Grossinger, Inner Traditions editorial
board member and cofounder and former publisher of North Atlantic Books. The
Sacred Planet collection, published under the umbrella of the Inner Traditions family
of imprints, includes works on the themes of consciousness, cosmology, alternative
medicine, dreams, climate, permaculture, alchemy, shamanic studies, oracles,
astrology, crystals, hyperobjects, locutions, and subtle bodies.

Note to the reader: *This book is intended to be an informational guide. The remedies,*
approaches, and techniques described herein are meant to supplement, and not to be a
substitute for, professional medical care or treatment. They should not be used to treat a
serious ailment without prior consultation with a qualified health care professional.

Cataloging-in-Publication Data for this title is available from the Library of Congress

ISBN 978-1-64411-608-1 (print)
ISBN 978-1-64411-609-8 (ebook)

Printed and bound in the United States by Versa Press, Inc.

10 9 8 7 6 5 4 3 2 1

Text design and layout by Virginia Scott Bowman
This book was typeset in Garamond Premier Pro and Gill Sans with Tide Sans and
Minion Pro used as display typefaces

To send correspondence to the author of this book, mail a first-class letter to the
author c/o Inner Traditions • Bear & Company, One Park Street, Rochester, VT
05767, and we will forward the communication, or contact the author directly at
www.Tara-Approach.org.

◆ ◆ ◆

This book is dedicated to the
Original Brilliance and
Embryonic Intelligence in everyone
and to its authentic emergence
at this turning point
for all humanity.

Contents

We are the bees of the invisible.

RAINIER MARIA RILKE

◆ ◆ ◆

At each state of its development, when it seems that an impasse has been reached, most improbably solutions have emerged that enabled the Earth to continue its development.

THOMAS BERRY

◆ ◆ ◆

Energy is not just oil and gas. Energy is an all-pervasive element of life. The broader our paradigm of energy, the wider our choices as human beings. Fossil fuels have fossilized our imagination, our potential, our creativity. We need to break free of this fossilization to choose life-enhancing pathways for ourselves, our species, and the planet.

VANDANA SHIVA

Foreword

By Cherionna Menzam-Sills, Ph.D.

As each of us forms in the womb, events occur that can have life-long effects. Despite, or perhaps because of its power, this essential time tends to hover in the shadows of our unconscious minds. It can take intention, focus, and therapeutic support to recover to consciousness the happenings and experiences of our earliest days.

During our time before birth, we form a physical body in which to navigate our world. In the process, we also form a brain and nervous system, along with a psyche. Seeds are planted and templates established for how we will interact with the life we are arriving into. Informed by the context we sense—even cellularly, as sperm, egg, and the original unicellular human we are when they unite—we prepare ourselves for the world our mother is carrying us into. Her perceptions of love, safety, and support or of isolation, toxicity, and threat affect our physical size, shape, and health, as well as our personality and behavioral and relational tendencies. The circumstances and emotions surrounding our conception and the discovery of the pregnancy are at least as significant in our formation as how we are born and received at birth. Any of these can be life enhancing or traumatic.

The field of epigenetics is demonstrating what many of us have intuitively known, that the experiences of our ancestors, even before our mother's also affects us. Our genes can be altered by our grandparents' traumas or lifestyle.

Embryology is not just about shaping physical structures. It also concerns perceptions, beliefs, and personal stories with which we emerge that equip us to meet life as we do. Attempting to heal ourselves can be thwarted without awareness of our prenatal life and the history of generations preceding us.

The Secret of Resilience is an intensely personal, beautifully poetic account of discovering and healing the effects of traumatic, embryological experience. Unlike most books on embryology, this one is spellbinding and hard to put down. Even for someone like me, who has been passionate about embryology and prenatal psychology since first encountering it in the early nineties, most embryology books are not this fascinating. Rarely are they this personal. But, in my experience, this has always been what Stephanie Mines is like!

Stephanie and I first met on our prenatal healing journey, guided by prenatal and birth therapy pioneer William Emerson, Ph.D. I remember holding Stephanie with some degree of awe as we dove in to our earliest traumas during a workshop held in the beautiful space of her studio in Eldorado Springs near Boulder, Colorado. As a graduate student discovering my own drive to learn more about embryology and pre- and perinatal psychology, I felt deeply touched and supported when Stephanie invited me to guest teach on this topic in her classes at Naropa Institute. She further supported my hungry inquiry by hosting my workshops in Embodying Embryology at her studio. It was natural for me to invite her in turn to be on my doctoral committee.

I can look back now and gratefully acknowledge Stephanie's persistent support when I was in the embryological stages of developing my own work in embryology and pre- and perinatal psychology. I wish all embryos could have such a generous, creative layer of support. But then, if Stephanie had been supported back in the womb as beautifully as she supported me in my work, she would not have birthed this remarkable book! As she herself elaborates, the work she offers has emerged out of her own suffering and challenges, starting before she was born.

Reading this latest book from Stephanie reminds me of the fiery passion I have perceived in her, which I suspect enabled her to survive not one but four attempts to abort her! My sense of awe continues! As we enter her story and those of other courageous individuals she has supported, we are invited to consider the profound effects of very early experience, beginning not only in the womb but even before as well. As Stephanie demonstrates through stories of her clients, our parents' experiences are carried epigenetically into our bodies and our psyches. Healing emerges within an accepting, listening field. Touch, via energetic bodywork, like the Art of Compassion Stephanie uses, enables the body to tell its story. Healing circles provide the safety needed for speaking what one remembers. Gathering information from parents and other ancestors can help complete a mysterious puzzle.

Stephanie describes how her awakening began with the birth of her first child, becoming a single mother, and being drawn intuitively to the energetic touch work of Mary Iino Burmeister. Her need to understand led her, against all odds, to graduate studies culminating in a doctorate in neuropsychology to understand the profound changes she witnessed through energy medicine. Along the way, memories of her own survival of abortion attempts and abuse as a child enabled her to enter a state of greater coherence, resilience, and health from which she could help facilitate others in their own healing. She describes her own and others' healing journeys as guided by her "prenatal being," holder of an "Embryonic Intelligence." In my own experience as a somatic pre- and perinatal and Biodynamic Craniosacral therapist, I similarly perceive the presence of what I call our original, embryological potential. As Stephanie notes, "Once liberated, Embryonic Intelligence will continually unfold, just as the embryo unfolds. It guides and we follow it, using our honed sensory acuity."

From this revived state of embryogenesis, we recognize our resonance with mother, including the Great Mother.

Stephanie's connection with nature, which she calls the Master Therapist, was clear to me back in the nineties as we gathered in her beautiful studio nestled in such natural beauty. Her story includes acknowledging the interconnectedness between us all and the planet—the Great Mother—we inhabit. The health of the Earth is intricately connected with our own, reminiscent of the relationship of mother to baby, via placenta, umbilical cord, and, after birth, the breast.

We need to heal the Earth as part of our own healing. As we heal ourselves and remember who we are, Mother Earth also heals. Indigenous cultures have always known this. It is time for us to remember. *The Secret of Resilience* is here to remind us who we are, who we have been, and who we have always been.

CHERIONNA MENZAM-SILLS, PH.D., began teaching Embodied Embryology through somatic movement in 1997 as part of her doctoral studies in pre- and perinatal psychology, which led to her teaching at Naropa University and the Santa Barbara Graduate Institute. She has taught and facilitated Pre- and Perinatal Psychology/Therapy, Continuum (a mindful movement practice), and Biodynamic Craniosacral Therapy internationally, often with her husband, biodynamics pioneer Franklyn Sills. Her background includes extensive study with pre- and perinatal psychology pioneers William Emerson and Ray Castellino and Continuum founder, Emilie Conrad, who authorized her to teach Continuum in 2007. Cherionna has authored two books, *The Breath of Life: An Introduction to Craniosacral Biodynamics* and, recently, *Spirit into Form: Exploring Embryological Potential and Prenatal Psychology*. Cherionna is committed in her work and life to embodied presence. You can learn more about Cherionna and her work at her website, **www.birthingyourlife.org**, and her online school with Franklyn Sills at **www.resourcingyourlife.org**.

Remembering the Future

All patterns of behavior have embryological developmental processes as their precursors. What we call instincts are the direct consequence of prenatal developmental events.

ERICH BLECHSCHMIDT

I REMEMBER MY FUTURE

Remembering starts with differentiation. Whereas differentiation is an organically natural process, in colonized societies it takes on another dimension. A multitude of forces accumulate to pry us apart from ourselves. These are the ones we must distinguish ourselves from to recall who we really are.

When you come in to the world without a sense of belonging it is only natural to search everywhere for that fulfillment. Some, like me, found fulfillment in groups built on outrage. Remembering is the only true antidote that I have found to endless cycles of trying to join, imitate, rescue—trying to do something. We are not meant to be followers. We are all meant to be leaders. I discovered this by truly remembering. Once I remembered my truth, it was easy and natural to remember my future.

It started spontaneously, long before I learned anything about neuroscience, energy medicine, or trauma. I was in my early thirties, the single mother of my first daughter, Sierra, living in San Francisco and facilitating a poetry program for the San Francisco Public Schools. Aside from the initiatory power of my first pregnancy and home birth, about which I had written a book, I knew nothing of embryology or psychology. What follows is excerpted from my journals written at that time, when I was living in San Francisco with my young daughter after I had separated from her father. I described an experience that went on for several days, culminating in the memory that my mother had made multiple attempts to abort me. My mother later confirmed that this was accurate. She had tried to abort me in the clumsy, brutal ways available to her then and wanting no one else to know what she was doing. Obviously, I survived.

Following is the excerpt from my journal.

A few days ago, out of nowhere, I felt acute pain in the area above my vagina. I was startled and panicked with worry. The sudden onset and the magnitude of the pain was impossible to ignore. Oddly my first reaction was to proceed to compulsively clean the house. Doing this allowed me, in ways I do not understand, to carry on and function, despite the pain. I cleaned until I had to race out to pick Sierra up from her play group. Once home I prepared food for us that I could not eat. The pain continued. I told Sierra that I was not feeling well and needed to rest. She came into the bedroom with me, bringing her crayons and drawing paper with her, snuggled up near me and began drawing. I closed my eyes. She was quite content. But I was in crisis, wondering how I could endure this discomfort and care for my child.

I had never felt anything like this before. It wasn't just the pain. Something else was going on. I seemed to be falling through layers of time and space. It wasn't dizziness. The only thing I had ever known that compared to this was labor. I curled into a fetal position. The pain was so intense that I could not restrain myself from moaning. With each moan, Sierra stroked my hair and told me about the princesses she was drawing, with stars in their hair. She tells me the princesses will make the pain go away. She crawls closer to me in the bed and holds me, cooing, "Poor baby—poor, poor baby." She rests her head on my shoulder, stretches out, and eventually falls asleep.

When she does, I crawl out of the bed carefully, so as not to disturb her. I have to vomit. I go into the bathroom and heave so much that I almost pass out. Then I have to poop, and massive elimination occurs, followed by more vomiting, more pooping, until I am exhausted. What is going on? Should I go to the hospital? How will I get there? I don't even have the capacity to call anyone. I surrender to my helplessness and the pain, the churning inside, and the weakness.

I lay down my yoga mat in my writing room and slowly ease into corpse pose. I fall into a kind of sleep, but my body is riddled with these waves of pain. I feel like I am drifting between planets, disconnected from my body, watching as if from outer space. My vagina pulses as if trying to deliver something. What is happening? I am terrified but incapable of doing anything.

Then the inside of my head fills with an amber light. I feel as if a being inhabits my torso, chin to belly, belly to chin. It is a huge golden egg. My arms and my legs rise up and hold the egg, barely able to encompass it. My veins feel as if they are carrying a fluid heavier and thicker than blood. I am inflamed, engorged. The pain intensifies. I cannot stifle the moans, though I do my best to subdue them. I do not want to wake my slumbering daughter.

Then somehow, I know that I am remembering something. I remember (don't ask me how) that my mother tried to abort me and that I am simultaneously remembering, in my body, her experience and my own. I am in an inner directed, spontaneous series of movements, cradling with love, the massive golden egg of who I am—the me that *aroused so much power and will that I survived. I know this in every cell of my body. There is no doubt.*

Then I hear something that sounds like instructions say this memory is an initiation. These are the words I record: "If everyone could remember, they would be in tune. There would be a cleansing and the confusion that oppresses humanity would dissolve. This has to be a slow process of remembering, but it will result in sweeping gestures of completion at just the right time. This is your work. It will bring peace and ease. You can carry this and deliver it. You already know how."

Now, forty years after this experience, its relevance for these times is clear. Indeed, these are the instructions I received to write this book.

1

Stepping onto the Path of the Wounded Healer

We are evolutionary inheritors of immense creativity and power.

TOM WINTON

We are not born with ego. Ego is compensatory for the loss of connection we endure. It is a strategy devised by the creative spirit that ultimately alchemizes everything into brilliant, purposeful expression, harmonious with and wedded to the web of life. When the illusion of disconnection is revealed, ego will be shed like the molting feathers of an eagle.

STEPHANIE MINES

I stepped onto the path of the Wounded Healer when I was conceived. From that moment I had an assignment. It was quite clear: take care of the others if you want to live. *Others* referred to literally everyone else around me, the whole world. I was designated as a Mother Tree. The clarity was sensory, cellular, and orienting. I have never veered from that path, though I shape-shift as I travel on it.

I begin this memoir with a tribute to the prenatal being who is still alive in me. I can see her quite clearly. She is absolutely incredible. She is pure—even pearl-like in her luminosity. She is astoundingly intelligent. This entire book is dedicated to her. Indeed, she is writing it.

She is the genius inside me who has never lost her confidence and clarity. She is a consciousness that has persevered despite all levels of threat to her life, including abuse and torture, horrendous, debilitating loss, and castigation. She directs these pages.

I surrender to the ongoing unfolding of her Original Brilliance, her regal directives initiated ages ago and passed down to her by countless ancestors. Now, when the fate of humanity is in question, I am acutely aware of how I come from ancient lineages of unity and inclusivity. I come from the lineages that protect the vulnerable—that have undying allegiance to the Earth and to all of nature. This is what it means to be a Mother Tree.

I listen to the voice of my prenatal self as I would listen to an oracle. She tells me that I have chosen to live in the era that signals the return of the powerful voices of these lineages that spawned me and of which I am an emanation. My prenatal life—indeed, virtually all my life experience—has been a rite of passage initiating me, over and over, on this path. It is humbling to see this.

I am, and always have been, an ecological being. From the moment of conception, I was intertwined with the web of life: metabolizing, refining, sorting, discarding, and fueling myself. I was shaped by where I was conceived, as well as by whom and when. The richness of sensory enmeshment mingled with my ecstatic and unyielding curiosity to evolve my original, utterly unique intelligence. The spirit of my determination transmuted the daunting odds of my circumstances and gave birth to my resilience. My intention in sharing this with you is to illuminate the path for your own remembering and model the courage for you to follow it as your destiny.

I was conceived on the southern border of the United States in Brownsville, Texas, at an army base. As I speak now, Brownsville is the site of a chaotic immigration crisis. I come from those who crossed and recrossed borders, repeatedly questing a safe haven that, more often than not, was denied. While my people have trod on countless roots, we have none. So, my conception in army housing in a place far from where my grandparents and extended family lived is not a surprise. Migration is almost my middle name.

Purity of being lives in the cells of our bodies like libraries of indigenous intelligence. This book models how to remember your wisdom and thereby live resiliently. This is my legacy, which I have come to these pages to transmit. Writing about it is also learning about it. Because this book is actually written by my prenatal self, it is an emergent unfolding. I am reading along with you.

SOUNDSCAPE

O my ancestors,
Give me the elixir of your love.
I search for it
In the embryology of my dreams.
I rise from your dark mineral waters
Singing jazz,
Moving in ways you have never seen.
I am loud and voluptuous.
I cannot be contained.
I am raucous.
I speak out of turn.
I break the rules.
I am the sperm and the egg.
I demolish the haunting with my poems.
You who were shuttered in the secrecy of pain,

Stripped of your wisdom,
Masquerading as white goyim,
I reveal you from where you were
Hidden from your own sight.
O my ancestors,
Give me the elixir of your love.
Let us drink it together,
Sit down to a meal,
Sleep in the same room,
Wake to see
Bright eyes delirious with reunion.
O my ancestors,
Bless me with your atonal incantations,
Liberate all the beautifully naughty children
Like me
Into their genius.
Let us clap our hands and shout,
Breathe in the pine scented air of our mountains,
Swim in the cool frothy waters of the
Rivers of Splendor
That regenerate our cells.

STEPHANIE MINES

Prenatal life is immersion in the living wisdom of our ancestors.

STEPHANIE MINES

By the twenty-second day in utero, and perhaps even before, sound is detected. All sound—the sounds of the mother's heartbeat, digestion, and breath, as well as all the surrounding sounds of the mother's environment. The development of the labyrinthian, cavelike structures of the ears (the oscillations of the fine hair cells in the organ of Corti) signal learning for the evolving being, who is comprehensively attuned to each opportunity to connect and communicate in the new world of form that is now home.

As I took in the episodic ebb and flow of my family's life, I, like you, oriented endearingly toward the people and the place that I now inhabited, albeit invisibly to them. They, however, were not invisible to me. The experiences of sound form a soundscape. My use of the word is inspired by conversations with my friend sound healer Clare Hedin and also from reading Dr. Alfred Tomatis and his protégé Paul Maudale's work.

My movements, and also the absence of movement, were directed and oriented by this soundscape. The word *orient* has a special meaning in relation to sound and hearing. The canals of the ears are regulators of balance and direction. The inner ear is the modulator of vestibular function. Sound, therefore, taught me about touch and movement. All my senses were infiltrated with the resonances of my soundscape. Where I went, how I got there, and how I felt in each position, all of these primary, early actions, my sweet, brilliant, prenatal self tells me, were orchestrated by my soundscape. Mine was a haunted soundscape, inundated by centuries of grief and horror. It was the soundscape of lifetimes of migration and loss. I took it in and vowed to serve that haunting, and, of course, courageous being that I am, I also vowed to liberate not only myself but also all those around me. This is not just the path of the Wounded Healer, it is the Heroine as Healer.

Each of us inhabits, imbibes, digests, and metabolizes the most interior intimacy of our family while we grow in utero. We hear and see the secrets, including all the secrets from the past. The uterus is like a cave of the ancestors. The egg that chose the sperm and made the union that resulted in personal form is a historian. The archives of lineage are implanted in the womb, and the conceptus absorbs those volumes, including the parts on audio.

What were the components of your soundscape? How did your soundscape influence your health, your relationships, and, actually, everything?

My earliest soundscape taught me that I had to focus. It was that or die. I inhabited a sound chamber of dissonance alternating with what seemed like endless silences punctuated by the vibrating plates of a steel bridge, echoing reverberation upon reverberation. These were the tuning forks of soma—the education of the soundscape self—and I was the patient listener, abandoned in the warm, toxic waves. My sonar antennae heard beyond sound, making me available for the messaging of birds and plants that spoke through my urban environment, along with the voices of time and the Earth. These composed a siren song of service, a plea for all children everywhere who were somehow one with me. I felt that calling through the soundscape, the echo chamber of my mother's womb.

Who Are You?

You are the one who
Folded and Unfolded
In rhythmic undulations
Perfectly timed
To orchestrate your dance of being.
You are the one who
Differentiated your cells
Separating and reforming
Ectoderm
Mesoderm
Endoderm.
You are the Director of Organogenesis.
You are the Initiator,
The one who understands everything
And therefore, forgives everything.

You wield the Sword of Apoptosis,
Remorselessly transitioning, discarding, evolving.
You are the Compass of the Sacred Directions,
Dorsal
Ventral
Cranial
Caudal.
You are the Germinator,
The One who Begins the Great Migrations:
The Ingression through the Primitive Streak,
The Voyage through the Womb.
You enticed your mother to build a placenta for you,
To surrender all her gateways,
And she complied.
You are the One Who Does Not Wait.
Because you know,
You act.

STEPHANIE MINES

2

Resilience and the Discovery of Original Brilliance

The door to this era's potential paradises is in hell.

REBECCA SOLNIT

When I met Mary Iino Burmeister, I was reeling from loss. My Wounded Healer's path, not yet even identified as such, was strewn with broken relationships, political activism gone awry, an interlude as a successful performing arts poet that scared me into retreat and disappearance, and the epiphanies of childbirth and motherhood. These latter two I found to be near-ecstatic experiences of love and surrender. I had just entered my thirties and had moved with my daughter to Sonoma County, having left San Francisco.

I was mysteriously resistant to success. I ran away from almost everything and everyone; I could not identify what I was running toward, though it might have been a vaguely defined fulfillment. I had no skill at prioritizing my own needs other than a drive to express myself, which I did primarily in poetry. I was a single mother with the daunting responsibility of caring for her small child while earning a living for us. I had come away from a raucous, destructive marriage. I was trying to follow a spiritual discipline as a way to define myself anew and claim the love I remembered. I thought that yoga and meditation, outlined by someone else, would return to me the union and beauty that was my inheritance. I kept mistakenly identifying fulfillment as following someone or something other than myself. I was a seeker without a center, a wildly expressive woman living like a hummingbird, flitting from one honeysuckle to another.

It is worth noting that Mary Iino Burmeister directed me to touch as a way of claiming selfhood—as a stimulus to unfolding authenticity. The self-care treatments she taught me, consisting of sequential holding on the sites I came to call sacred, were like homeopathic doses of self-love. I became devoted to the practice and still am. It answers the unnamed need of the generous, forgiving, caring, creative prenatal self who is me—the embryonic me.

Mary Iino Burmeister opened a portal to my capacity to evolve through touch—my touch, not someone else's. It seemed magical, but at the same time it was completely ordinary. It was thoroughly somatic. Using the map of the body that Mary provided and her scant directives about how to touch the sites, I began to change in ways that surprised me and that were clearly positive.

Most remarkable of all, in this evolution I remembered my Original Brilliance. This was not a thought or a plan. It was behavior, action, manifestation. I was freed to be spontaneous. I stopped feeling ashamed and embarrassed about my unique expression and started enjoying it. The only thing that was different in my difficult life of working, earning money, caring for a child by myself, and squeezing my poetry writing into the middle of the night or the wee hours of the morning was that I was touching myself. I was being restored back to who I was at the moment I took form—back to that incredible light force of a being who had survived death threats and whom I can now claim as myself. This,

I can say now, is the Path of Resilience. Resilience truly and enduringly arises when we remember ourselves.

Back

We are calling you back
The birds trill
On a shrouded Northwest
Morning
When I am
Listening.
Ancient trees
Like Masai
Surround me.
For this moment
It does not appear that
The world is coming to an end.
There are no lying politicians in the forest.
Silence, the robe of my Mother,
Soothes my brain into
Believing
There is nothing for me to do.
Wearing pajamas, hair wild,
I am welcome
Without doubt;
Reminded of when
I knew I was meant to be here,
Back when
Time was an endless scroll of love;
Back when space was pure possibility.
What infirmities we create
In order to find our way
Back

To the vastness
Where the birds that speak to me
Recover from their flights.

STEPHANIE MINES

THE ART OF COMPASSION

Embryology is the study of creation and creation is not just
the beginning. It is the ongoing ever-present energy that
assumes patterns in the body with each present moment.

MARY IINO BURMEISTER

Mary Iino was born in 1920 in the Pacific Northwest of the United States, where I now live. In fact, as I write these words, I am on a train moving toward the city where she was born. She was a Nisei, and her parents were proud of their heritage and also of their success in the United States. When they were interned during World War II, the shock was unfathomable. At her first opportunity an enraged and outraged Mary headed for Japan, vowing never to return to the United States. At the age of twenty-two, Mary met Jiro Murai, who taught her the Art of Compassion. Almost five years later she met Gil Burmeister, whom she married and with whom she returned to the United States, with the blessing and encouragement of Jiro Murai. In her new iteration as a wife, and then as a mother, Mary continued her studies with Jiro Murai by correspondence.

When I met Mary nothing in my conscious mind and none of the practical circumstances of life for me and my little family of mother and daughter would suggest that I was about to enter an apprenticeship in the healing arts. I had no conscious desire to do so. A series of circumstances literally placed me on this path, almost against my will. I stumbled awkwardly into this apprenticeship, but eventually it took hold of me in a way that I seemed incapable to resist. I followed the unfolding of my evolving self with incredulity and even delight at times. Though I felt inadequate, misaligned, doubtful, and skeptical, I was, at the same time, magnetized into what would become a meeting with myself.

It is only by looking backward now that I see the benevolence of how I was seduced into resilience and the path of the Wounded Healer. It was a purely somatic seduction. I was pulled onto this path by my evolution in the direction of health, like a flower turning toward the sun. How many powerful ancestors must have been involved in these logistics?

I followed Mary as a teacher for more than twenty years, despite barely having the resources to do so. Every day, without fail and continuing to this present moment, I use what she taught me about touch and the map of the body, which I have now named the Map of the Sacred Sites. No matter what else happens, I continue the self-care Mary introduced me to, often merging it with writing and dance.

As someone who had lived with the constrictions of intense self-criticism, unraveling of myself from that incessant entrapment became a heuristic, motivational force. My intelligence and curiosity were tantalized by what was happening to me, and after I began sharing the Art of Compassion with others, I saw straightaway their overwhelmingly positive responses.

At this point in my life, I already had two degrees. My undergraduate studies had been in literature and my masters was in creative writing, all earned before my daughter was born. My dream for myself had always been the writer's life. Yet this inner unraveling was opening me to the world of science, which I had never considered, and this world seemed to have more dimension than the writer's life. A different destiny was forming even as I moved toward it, with my curiosity—the hallmark quality of my embryonic, prenatal self—in the lead.

This led me eventually to pursue a doctorate so that I could understand what was happening to me and to the others with whom I shared the practice. How did the body and the mind work together? What were the sites, and why did touching them make so much difference in feeling, movement, gesture, voice quality, health, and all behavior? How could touching these sites so efficiently lessen pain? And how did my experiences of abuse, trauma, and shock play roles in shaping nervous system responses? Was this individuated or generalized? How was it that wholeness was now emerging for me through the simple acts of self-touch?

People living with distressing symptoms that medical doctors had no answers to were drawn to the informal classes I taught, and they also found themselves making breakthroughs to wholeness. I invented internships for myself, like volunteering at a nursing home, where I watched while elderly people who were uncomfortable and restricted in their bodies eased out of constriction and into relaxation.

One incident during this period stopped me in my tracks. My neighbor had a six-year-old grandson with cerebral palsy. I occasionally helped her out by babysitting him. One afternoon while Grandma ran errands, I practiced holding sequences on some of the sacred sites on him, and he changed before my eyes from a contorted, distressed child to a happy one, at ease with himself. When Grandma returned, she was awe-struck. Michael had never before looked so soft and content. Of course, I had to teach her how to help her sweet boy, the abandoned child of her crack-addicted son and his wife. She was profoundly grateful, and our friendship deepened.

I could not allow myself to ignore or take lightly the accumulation of these experiences. I was weaving them into a fabric of possibility. They were inspiring me—lifting me out of the isolation and self-consciousness that were habituated and limiting. I was waking to a sense of newness and anticipation each day. I felt enthusiastic about what I, despite all my many imperfections, could offer others who were suffering in a variety of ways, including in manners very similar to mine because of our shared developmental struggles in dysfunctional homes.

The hope was tantalizing. I became preoccupied with it. I began searching for doctoral programs that might somehow encompass these questions, that might offer some direction to my contemplations and fill in the blanks in Mary's koanlike teachings. Neuroscience and neuropsychology came the closest to meeting my needs, and once that was clarified doors opened to allow me to move in that direction, even as a single, working mother. I was exhilarated. This was a breakthrough. I could suddenly envision a different future for my child and myself—one in which I might have a career that would make our lives much more comfortable. In addition, the possibility that I could be an instrument to alleviate suffering was something of such magnitude that it was close to a spiritual awakening. I was going beyond what I had learned from Mary, but she had planted the seed of possibility with her resources and her faith in human potential.

It would take at least a decade from the day I met Mary for me to identify the origins of what Mary taught as the channels of the Extraordinary Vessels or what I now call the Rivers of Splendor. These are the conduits of resilience that fuel prenatal life. This required study, research, contemplation, and consultation with others. Ultimately this meant completing my doctorate, doing postdoctoral studies with Peter Levine and others, and being of service to thousands and thousands of people. It required clinical trials and meticulously tracking the transformational processes that moved individuals out of traps of pain and constriction, self-loathing and limitation, loneliness and isolation, insecurity, and self-hatred toward wholeness, expanded consciousness, and connection to the Earth. All of this directed me to the treasures that are within the Rivers of Splendor.

These vessels of resilience are our birthright. The climate crisis, which is written in Code Red, a high alert for humanity, trumpets the necessity to make such wisdom broadly available. As the trauma specialist I have become I can say that bringing these resources to a level of groundswell, globally and universally, can and will make the difference between life and death for communities, for vulnerable populations, and for all people. This is the mission of my brilliant, loving prenatal self. She basks in this delivery. This book explains the relationship between resilience and Original Brilliance, woven into my personal unfolding and that of others whom I have had the privilege to know.

3
The Way of the Great Physician
Transmuting Poison to Medicine

The Great Physician

The Great Physician
Is she who knows
The metallurgy of grief.
She transmutes vilification,
Betrayal,
Scapegoating,
Gaslighting,
Torture,
Finger-pointing,
Blaming,
Castigation,
And all manner of ignorance
Into enthusiasm for the future of humanity.
As truth rises to the surface of my body,
Bones mend, tendons reknit,
Joints ease, and

Resilience arises.
Heart feeds mind poems,
Healthcare strategies and
The architecture of leadership.
The Great Physician breathes the
Recipe for making poison into medicine.
This is the Destiny of Fulfillment.

STEPHANIE MINES

TRAUMATIC REPETITION: FOOTPRINTS OF EMBRYOGENESIS

Whatever is implicitly initiated and practiced by the body
during its early development is enacted at a later date.

ERICH BLECHSCHMIDT

What if I told you that everything from your taste in food to your taste in partners is a reflection of the experiences and sensations from so early in your life that you have no cognitive memory of them?

If you are curious enough about this, I will go on to say that the way you walk, your weight and your gait, your posture, the way you sleep and lean, your gestures, and the tone of your voice are all derived from the sensations and events known only to you from when you were a tiny being.

The intelligence, creativity, curiosity, and vitality that motivates you now motivated you with significantly greater force when you were much smaller. Furthermore I would say, if you are still listening, that reclaiming the awareness that infused you then is the key not only to personal fulfillment but also to the continuity of humanity. In this unprecedented era that exposes the underbelly of our ignorance, the secrets of alchemizing intelligence that you harbor are needed and will emerge, just as the veins on the hands of elders reveal the rich indigo of their blood.

My prenatal experiences of entering, at conception, a world in which I instantaneously felt I did not have a place was replicated in how I entered everything that followed, including the world of learning the Art of Compassion from Mary Iino Burmeister. This pattern marked all my beginnings until the writing of this book.

I became quite ill during my first class with Mary, just as I was, unbeknownst to my family, extremely unwell in utero. I was born with lung afflictions that became severe, life-threatening bronchial pneumonia shortly after birth. As I matured these tendencies morphed into extreme respiratory vulnerability, acute sensitivity to environmental toxins, and chronic and severe asthma.

In all the classes I attended with Mary, despite how I felt, I stayed focused on her every word. I hunkered down with a notebook in the back or in a corner of the room and listened, watched, and wrote. In so doing, unbeknownst to me, I was alchemizing—transmuting the feeling of alienation and unwantedness into purpose. I embodied the scribe, and my attention was riveted on the task of taking accurate and clear notes. I used my stenographer's skill, cultivated in summer school classes when I was in high school because I knew I would have to be able to do something practical to earn a living. I had a way of staying on track with my documentation long before computers.

Mary was a diminutive, perfectly attired woman who strode, bright-eyed and determined, toward the podium from which she taught. She wore stiletto heels that clicked sharply on the floor, drawing us to the color coordination of wide belts with matching shoes that were almost like a uniform. This belt and high heels ensemble disappeared after the accident that ended her teaching and changed not only her footwear but her entire demeanor as well.

In all the early classes with Mary that I attended, I was preoccupied with worry that I might lose the employment from which I had requested time off. Those jobs were the only source of income for me and my daughter. Could I survive and learn? Could I survive and follow my instincts? Could I survive and fulfill my responsibilities? These were the questions that haunted my entire existence and that were amplified by the megaphone of new beginnings. I know now these feelings to be echoes from the womb. Yet even then, before I had the language, I was dissolving my worry with my determination to show up. I gave myself no credit for this. In fact, I berated myself for being so irrational as to take time off from a paying job to do something for which there was no clear outcome other than preserving the pursuit of curiosity. I was not yet an alchemist or a metallurgist.

On my own, after the classes, in whatever time I could find, I became a self-proclaimed and daring investigative scientist, testing new formulas. As a working mother with no social life, I could follow a discipline of practicing all the touch combinations that Mary taught. I was aware that I was changing as a result of the practices and that they were drawing me to interior investigations that were revelatory. I was becoming someone I had not yet met. The alchemical brew was bubbling. I was tracking it, documenting it, but I had no idea that I was on the path of the Great Physician, the Wounded Healer, and the Metallurgist of Grief.

Recollections spewed out of me and were reformatted as I gently held the sites on my body. I was the witness of the deeply buried emotions I had secreted away. Alongside the sexual and physical abuse in my early life, there were the scenes from my radical political activism, the years of daring protest, and the retribution I received from all fronts, as well as the violent, romantic relationships that seemed to trail me like my own shadow. I reviewed and rewrote these experiences, transcribing the physical, emotional, and psychic imprints and then reframing them, seeing them as patterns, and taking responsibility for them, leaving my victimhood behind. These were the rituals to which I apprenticed myself to end traumatic repetition. I created them independently, with no therapeutic guidance, in a fluid unfolding from my somatic process. And they worked.

THE WOUNDED HEALER LINEAGE OF
THE ART OF COMPASSION

Mary was the first to name in English and record what Jiro Murai, her teacher, had excavated from his mysterious morphogenic resonance with the Earth beneath him as he lay on his deathbed. At the age of twenty-seven he was dying of leukemia, alone in a mountain cabin, when he spontaneously began to put his hands into postures and touch areas of his body until, after chills and fevers, he recovered and emerged to devote his life to what he had been graced to experience. This was the source from which flowed what Mary taught me.

Jiro Murai had been a renegade who outcast himself from his family's professional physician status. The profligate second son became terminally ill and returned home to die. The disease process reduced him to the most surrendered state of receptivity, and there, one could say, he encountered the possibility of reclaiming his own Original Brilliance. Gratitude motivated Jiro Murai to devote his life to uncovering the healing process that had brought him back to himself. When Mary met him, he was already a wisdom holder, and as such he recognized her as his disciple.

Mary taught regularly in Santa Rosa when I was living near there. Her programs were organized by one of her first students, Pamela Markarian Smith. The two women had a very strong bond. Pamela became my teacher as soon as I met her, which was at that first class with Mary, so whenever Mary returned, I was more and more prepared to understand her. Eventually I became Pamela's apprentice, so when Mary taught in Santa Rosa, I could tag along on their personal visits. It felt amazing to me to be included in their company. It was as if a curse had been lifted and I was momentarily freed from banishment.

Pamela invited me to stay in her home the summer before I moved to Colorado, while my daughter was visiting her father. I worked alongside her every day. It was a treasured opportunity for mentorship from Mary's most advanced disciple and protégé. Pamela had a thriving practice, and I was her assistant, pairing with her for every session and following her directions. Simultaneously she explained why she had selected the treatments she chose. She pointed out to me the patients' subtle shifts in skin and voice tone, posture, and gestures. Pamela was tutoring me about where to look to identify how each individual's energy was shifting. In the evenings and on the weekends, we would discuss the treatments, with Pamela giving me the backstory to the energetic dynamics that were evolving and the methodology behind their success. It was my personal graduate school, and I was humbled to be so fortunate, even if I did not have a clue about where all this was going.

Pamela was a tall, dark-haired, exotic, and willowy beauty. Heads turned when she walked by. She had a career as an actress and a model before she became extremely ill with respiratory conditions, similar to the ones with which I struggled. She discovered Mary in Southern California and grew to be deeply loyal to her because she felt that what Mary taught her had saved her life. Pamela gave up all aspirations for stardom so that she could immerse herself in what Mary transmitted to her. It was her entire world. She studied continuously. It was humbling, and even baffling to me, that she selected me to learn from her in such proximity.

I moved to Boulder, Colorado, from Northern California to start anew. I wanted a change from the California ambience. I chose Boulder, in part, because Mary taught there, at the Rolf Institute, founded by chiropractor and innovative healer Ida Rolf. The Rolf Institute was at the end of a tree-lined residential neighborhood nestled at the foot of the Flatirons. The sharp, serrated landscape of snow-covered peaks embracing a village of industrious, innovative thinkers and entrepreneurs, spiritual seekers, and poets was near magical for me. Perhaps I had finally made a good decision? Maybe I was in the right place?

I got a job working as an administrative assistant for an herbal company. When the Rolf Institute advertised for someone to help out on the weekends, I jumped at the chance. This gave me an insider's view of the cadre of Mary's students, many of whom were Rolfing students and practitioners.

I had a small basement apartment within walking distance of the Rolf Institute. Outside my door were winding trails traversing the rolling hills and deep valleys of the Dakota Ridge. My daughter was enrolled in a good school. She found friends that she soon preferred to me. This left me space for more study and practice and to investigate the possibility of finding a graduate program that would answer my questions. I built myself a folding treatment table. I had visions of one day having a practice like Pamela's, though my only patient was my daughter.

By now I had a near-obsessive fascination with the inner workings of the human nervous system, just from using my own as my laboratory. I detailed everything I was experiencing in notebooks that I reviewed as if seeking a missing puzzle piece. Graduate program or not, I defined myself as a student, and that identity felt completely comfortable—even comforting. The practices were birthing something within me that was unfamiliar—a sense of well-being. The Main Central Vertical Flow, in particular, gave me a palpable experience of having a midline, a central channel, and something new—an anchor.

MY STRANGE LOVE AFFAIR

Eventually Mary remarked each time she saw me enter a class that "it wouldn't be a class without you." Apparently, I repeated the classes more than other students and became a familiar face, despite hiding at the

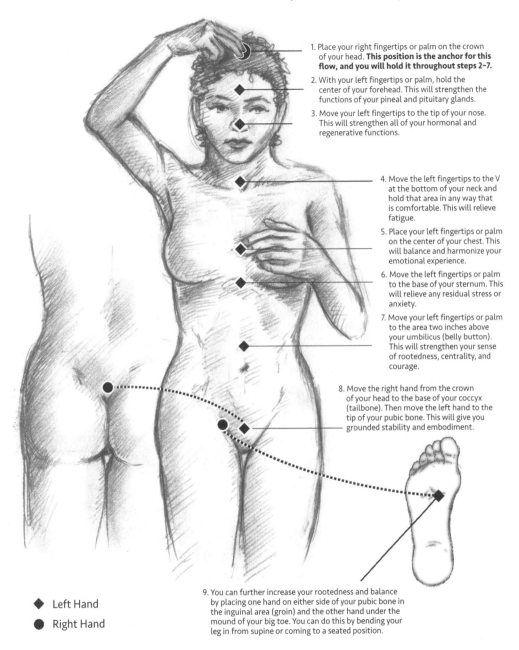

1. Place your right fingertips or palm on the crown of your head. **This position is the anchor for this flow, and you will hold it throughout steps 2–7.**

2. With your left fingertips or palm, hold the center of your forehead. This will strengthen the functions of your pineal and pituitary glands.

3. Move your left fingertips to the tip of your nose. This will strengthen all of your hormonal and regenerative functions.

4. Move the left fingertips to the V at the bottom of your neck and hold that area in any way that is comfortable. This will relieve fatigue.

5. Place your left fingertips or palm on the center of your chest. This will balance and harmonize your emotional experience.

6. Move the left fingertips or palm to the base of your sternum. This will relieve any residual stress or anxiety.

7. Move your left fingertips or palm to the area two inches above your umbilicus (belly button). This will strengthen your sense of rootedness, centrality, and courage.

8. Move the right hand from the crown of your head to the base of your coccyx (tailbone). Then move the left hand to the tip of your pubic bone. This will give you grounded stability and embodiment.

9. You can further increase your rootedness and balance by placing one hand on either side of your pubic bone in the inguinal area (groin) and the other hand under the mound of your big toe. You can do this by bending your leg in from supine or coming to a seated position.

◆ Left Hand

● Right Hand

Figure 3.1. Main Central Vertical Flow Exercise

This self-care treatment can be done most easily from a supine position (lying on your back). You can use any portion of it for its expressed purposes alone, shorten the flow if you do not have time for all of it, or do the entire sequence at once. For each step, hold the positions until you feel a sense of balance, relief, or completion. Trust your experience.

back. Still, I felt like a beginning student and an outsider. I was intent on finding my way through the labyrinthine, theoretical structures of Mary's teachings that I was sure others were grasping easily. I would not stop until I fully grokked them. That was my commitment. My self-care treatments were a sanctuary. These were reassuring interludes, awakening authentic respiration, elongation, and a wellspring of refreshment. It was my self-care experience that interrupted the habitual refrains that there was something wrong with me and that I needed to be fixed. This began to be countered by a new song, one that was composing itself anew every day, about who I was and what was possible in my life.

As I continued, self-treatments further muted tortuous mental agitation and silenced relentless nervous system discord. My mind-body found an evolving and miraculous peace that supported my spiritual practices, sense of humor, resilience, parenting skills, and poetry. So, I returned over and over to Mary, hoping, or even anticipating, that hearing her one more time would crystallize the system for me. I pored over the few texts Mary provided. This kept me company during long Colorado winters when I was snowed in and on beautiful springtime nights when my mind sought company. Each season now was affiliated with what Mary was teaching me about the elements. I understood my passion for the exquisite autumns in the foothills of the Flatirons as an expression of my healing need. The delicious summers when couples strolled entwined with each other tortured me—the single mother chained to a relentless work schedule and unceasing demand.

A remarkable kinship with the Sacred Sites resulted. I began to think of them as my dearest companions. I could not speak of this to anyone lest they think I was crazy. This worsened the stress I felt about parenting alone. I had no one to consult with or advise me about this and no model from which to draw. I was frequently troubled and distraught about how to handle situations and meet expenses. The only comrades I found who listened deeply to me, who had the patience and attention to hear me out, who commiserated with me and sought to comfort me, and who actually presented me with solutions through the vehicle of my own being were the Sacred Sites—though I had not yet coined that term for them. They were my lovers and my friends.

Little did I know I was carrying forward an ageless wisdom of communing with the invisible and transmuting poison to medicine. I was not thinking about the embryonic me or even the small child me who wove threads of hope out of the unknown. Embryology was not yet part of my formulations, and I was ignorant of theories of attachment and neurodevelopment. I was simply, independently, following my sensation where it directed me. I was being my embryonic self, and it felt very good.

I somehow managed to scrape together the funds to undertake regular intensive treatments with Mary in Scottsdale, Arizona, where she lived and had an office. Each of these periods was immersion in a sea of energetic change. I wandered through these times in the strange upscale land of Scottsdale, where I really felt like an alien. Yet inevitably I awoke to a new clarity, radiant with presence, usually within a few days after my return home.

This all led, quite organically, to providing treatments for others and teaching self-care courses to small groups of curious people who somehow found me. I never advertised or took any steps to create a business, but others who were drawn to new ways of experiencing their full potential and who were struggling with mysterious afflictions, such as mine, were drawn to me. Mary often spoke of this natural process as the way she had begun to share the Art of Compassion, so I felt reassured in this unfolding. It was a signal I was part of a lineage that was serving me just as I hoped to serve others.

The practice of documenting treatment outcomes that I had established for myself now was used as well for the sessions I was asked to provide for others. Buttressed by what I gleaned from my apprenticeship with Pamela Markarian Smith, I created a research model that I would return to later when I did clinical trials and that I would eventually teach to my students. I charted my observations, the changes my clients reported, and nuanced shifts in bioelectrical sensation. I was determined to find the link between rhythmic and textural reports in pulse and parallel shifts in consciousness and behavior. I was on the lookout for what I, independent of any study or guidance, was beginning to identify as traumatic repetition and intergenerational trauma, though I did not yet have that language. I was on my own with these formulations. Mary was clear that she was not a psychologist and that her sense of psychology was only what she called the five attitudes: worry, fear, anger, grief, and pretense.

I was becoming a scientist and a writer of a different sort from what I had first hoped to be. I became a journalist of alchemical transmutation in the minds and bodies of people afflicted by difficult, sometimes horrific, and always overwhelming experiences. It was notable to me how many people had been sexually abused—how many had emotional abuse in their backgrounds, regardless of demographics. I posited the social and political ramifications of what I was observing and looked to the systemic conditions that had manipulated all of us so that we were left with an insistent need to uncover our personal truth.

4
Beyond Epigenetics

We are born out of ourselves.

JAAP VAN DER WAL

Continuing to use my body and my biography as my laboratory, I took on the themes of traumatic repetition and intergenerational trauma by reviewing the patterns of my life and how they resembled, or differed from, what I knew about my family, especially my mother. It is noteworthy that my investigations into epigenetics started before I entered my doctoral studies. There were very few books or studies about epigenetics, and certainly none in popular parlance. I did not even know that word. Neither Mary nor anyone in the communities of her students were discussing trauma, much less inherited trauma. Despite the trauma that Mary and Pamela had experienced, they never made those references, nor did they suggest a connection between trauma and the healing process.

What was occurring for me was arising completely from within myself. I mention this because it is, in part, what assures me of the viability of a groundswell of Regenerative Health awakening. If these insights can arise from me in response to energetic recalibration and shifts in my nervous system, they can happen for you and for anyone. I have seen this to be true, time and time again, when the resources are available. The stories later in this book point to this.

Everyone in my family, it seemed, lived in reaction to my father. He was the catalyst for a life of terror and hyper-vigilance, sending us reeling from his extreme actions, whether when he was with us or when he abandoned us. But the person who shaped our lives on a constant continuum was my mother. I could not ignore the fact that I, like my mother much of the time, was the mainstay, the only stable adult in a single-parent household.

ENDING TRAUMATIC REPETITION

I was a single mother as my own mother had been. What my lived experience revealed, daily, was that this was an extremely complex emotional, psychological, and physiological lifestyle. It was rigorous, demanding, and nonstop. There was no downtime—no respite. Basically, a single mother runs a marathon every day of her life. I don't think there is anything else quite like it. I frequently had to take on additional jobs to make ends meet, and even doing that I sometimes needed financial assistance along with supplemental food stamps and other welfare services. I found this demeaning and shameful, but I had no choice. I know that my mother had experienced these same strains, not because she talked about them but because I witnessed her and sensed what she did not share.

My father had an undiagnosed head injury and likely was an alcoholic, and I eventually discovered that he was also a bigamist. He disappeared for long periods of time, months that often turned into years, and then would return unexpectedly. There would be strange phone calls as a precursor to his reappearance, chilling series of heavy breathing and stumbling words, call after call—the signals of his dreaded return. Until finally, one day, he disappeared completely. When he died, another family, one we never met, received whatever benefits he was due from his military service and social security payments.

My mother had only a high school education and struggled to find jobs that would sustain her and her two children. She found her comfort and release in watching television. She did not interact with me very much or ask me about myself. She was totally drained at the end of every day. I felt her enormous grief and exhaustion and wanted, more than anything else, to assuage it, which I did by earning money from odd jobs and trying to keep the house clean and take care of my brother. Otherwise, I kept to myself as much as possible, consuming literature, writing, and going on long walks that usually ended at a library.

I was in the single mother trap when I met Mary Iino Burmeister, worrying almost constantly about money. Unlike my mother, though, I could not squelch my creative and expressive needs. Writing poetry and short stories, dance, and all the things I treasured and needed as much as food or sleep were squeezed into the last few moments that I could sequester from my single-parent life. Still, I was acutely aware I had mirrored my mother's dilemma through my own traumatic repetition of choosing an unsupportive father for my child, leaving me as the primary provider and family mainstay, all the while feeling completely unqualified. It is a nerve-racking place to be.

Holding the Sacred Sites in various combinations when I was alone was the beginning of a hope that I might find a real, physiological route out of traumatic repetition and intergenerational trauma. Writing poetry, journaling, movement, and reading had long sustained me, but they had not made a physiological difference. It was suddenly quite clear to me that without somatic, physiological, nervous system–based reprogramming that arose authentically from within me, real transformation was not possible. At least not for me. I felt like I had found the key to liberation, and it was dangling in front of me, sparkling and tantalizing.

It was as if I were redirecting the current in my body so that it flowed upstream instead of downstream with each application. This resulted in sustained shifts; in fact, the results accumulated. Whereas the weight of all that I juggled before had burdened me, now the juggling itself became playful. My metabolism shifted so that I experienced expanded cycles of endurance, adding waking hours to each day. It was as if I suddenly discovered pockets of time I did not realize were there and emptied them into an elasticized version of each day, with moments expanding even as I inhabited them.

The rhythms of my being changed as I awakened the Sacred Sites. Later, when I studied epigenetics, I realized that I had been carrying in my biorhythms the echoes of my mother's despair as well as the turbulence of my entire lineage, particularly my father. In my deep interactions with the Sacred Sites, I unearthed my own rhythms. These were the dominant, originating rhythms of my beautiful, creative spirit and the rhythms of the prenatal being who inhabited the biofields of my ancestry and took form so as to be of service. These were the individuated, differentiated rhythms of my being and not the rhythms of a person or a culture outside of me.

The pulsations that I titrated as I listened to them in each site and on my wrists as I became more and more confident with pulse-listening were the direct feedback about my rhythmic evolution. I could track bioelectric pulsation from day to day and even from hour to hour. I could see, hear, and feel, by reading the bioelectrical pulses in the sites and on my wrists, what was happening to me energetically. I perfected the art of sensory acuity as I brought forward my true nature. I tracked my senses home to myself. The sites guided me, but it was me who was awakening.

Just as time emerged like flowers blooming out of hidden cracks in each day, so did my understanding of the Art of Compassion. The mysteries of what I learned from Mary and Pamela became clear for me in the context of the resolution of trauma and shock. Even before I returned to graduate school, I was piecing together patterns of nervous system disrepair and recalibration and formulating theories about the interface between energy and neurophysiology.

It would take additional research and learning for me to realize that the Sacred Sites act to regulate the flow of the Rivers of Splendor, but that is what was happening and long before I could name it. My nervous system was shedding the corrosive layers of trauma I had acquired. The Sacred Sites were doing their job of restoring my essence. As Yvonne Farrell says in her book *Psycho-Emotional Pain and the Eight Extraordinary Vessels,* "Although someone may feel lost, those feelings and the suffering associated with them in no way damages who they are at the core. The Eight Extraordinary Vessels remind us of the uniqueness and perfection of our original self, and they allow us to once again bring forth the light that is our purpose for being here. They put us back on track to pursuing our destiny."

That is exactly what happened. It evolved so organically I could not see it coming. Traumatic repetition was ending in my nervous system as habituated neuronal consolidation dissolved and unforeseen, unpredictable options presented themselves. As I found equilibrium and self-respect I opened to the unforeseen and emergent opportunities that I could now recognize and welcome. Mary spoke often about how inner and outer reality mirror each other. As a philosophical statement, that is tantalizing and seductive. As a lived experience, it is the miracle of transformation. For me, it was the Metallurgy of Grief.

With this same natural unfolding, the graduate program I longed for appeared as the result of some synchronistic conversations with people I encountered, one of whom was José Argüelles. José, author of *The Mayan Factor,* lived not far from me. His wife also studied with Mary. José was on the faculty of Union Institute. He opened the doors that made it possible for me, single working mother or not, to return to school and explore the probing questions that begged me for their answers, night and day.

The doctoral program was initiatory for me. My burgeoning scientific mind met my poet's heart, and the two aspects of myself found a way to embrace. I prioritized the incubation of my ideas. I had to keep earning a living, so I developed an extremely rigorous and strict schedule that, to my amazement, was liberating.

THE PATH OF THE
WOUNDED HEALER IS REVEALED

I was pleased, of course, when I was invited to participate in the first ever advanced courses Mary taught. In these classes Mary offered, without fanfare, material previously unavailable. She exposed more of the storehouse of wisdom she retained in her consciousness and memory from her studies with Jiro Murai. It was in these classes that she referred, albeit only by inference, never explicitly, to the relationship between prenatal, embryonic life and the fundamental structure of the Art of Compassion. Mary had seen some of my early writing in my doctoral process and was pleased with the direction my research was taking. I had not yet landed on the focus of traumatic brain injury that was to shape my internship, research, and thesis, but Mary would learn of that, and nod her approval, before the tragic injury that changed everything.

I was traveling to attend what would be the last of these classes when Mary fell in her own home and endured a head injury. After that she never taught again. Paradoxically, it was her disappearance as a resource that led me to solve the puzzle of how this medicine worked. Losing my teacher jump-started a leap forward on my path as a Wounded Healer. The irony and the beauty that my doctoral research was an investigation of traumatic brain injury, such as the one that took my teacher from me, and that this was also what had damaged my father and thereby stole my childhood, does not escape me.

Looking back at this circuitous journey I still am in awe at how I managed, despite overbearing doubt and insecurity, to find the jewel buried in the middle of the labyrinth—the one that oddly enough seemed to be waiting there for me. That jewel, the source of resilience, is what is unfolding for you here, in this book, because the time has come for everyone to partake of this medicine. Mary's most often quoted phrase, "Be the star you are," I now know for certain speaks to *the secret of resilience* and the Rivers of Splendor as the conduits of that secret. That star truth is most decidedly what magnetized my astute prenatal self to this path and took me beyond epigenetics.

5

All Rivers of Splendor
Flow to the Sea

Embrace these vessels and your destiny unfolds.

Yvonne Farrell

I created the TARA Approach for the Resolution of Shock and Trauma once it was clear to me that what I had learned about neurodevelopment matched, albeit in a different language, what Mary taught. The Rivers of Splendor, known as the Extraordinary Vessels or Meridians in other systems, clear the neuronal pathways of the Wounded Healer for the evolution of consciousness. That evolution, and the resilience that accompanies it, began from the moment I first touched the Sacred Sites. I propelled it forward by nurturing it with my inner awakenings, carefully charted to solve the puzzles of my existence and claim my Embryonic Intelligence.

Mary was unable to evolve her teachings any further after her accident. At almost exactly the same time huge swaths of the global population and the medical world were reeling from the AIDS epidemic. I was poised at a new threshold. I had successfully completed my doctorate and shortly thereafter established a private practice that rapidly flourished.

The parallels between that time and now are so many that they could be the topic of another book. Suffice it to say for now that a global epidemic gave sway to the TARA Approach for the Resolution of Shock and Trauma. In just the same way this book was triggered by my response to the climate crisis and the global pandemic that is tied to it—this synchronicity is not random.

I was compelled by strong, guiding, somatic inner forces to bring my fusion of neuroscience and energy medicine forward and be of service during the AIDS epidemic. Alongside that decision the name for it emerged: TARA (Tools for Awakening Resources and Awareness) declared herself, like a child at the moment of discovery, with a nod to the Buddhist concept of Tara who, like Kwan Yin, is considered the embodiment of mercy. The TARA Approach was ignited by people whose lives were on the line. This was as close as I could come to merciful service. That choice echoes loudly again right now as all of humanity is under similar threat.

The AIDS epidemic and my services to the people living with AIDS further deepened and illuminated my investigations into the specific relationships between trauma and immune function. Virtually all the people I served who were living with HIV and AIDS had experienced unrelenting trauma and shock. Most of them had histories of suffering from prejudice, racism, body dysmorphia, exclusion, sexual and physical violence, isolation, alienation, emotional abuse, poor medical service, addiction and the punitive treatment of addiction, disempowerment, and dehumanization. I, and those I trained to be TARA practitioners and teachers at this time, tended to these courageous people in life and death. We listened to their stories, traced what happened to their T cells as trauma was resolved, tracked the evolution of their symptoms, and sat by their deathbeds.

One of my foremost students at that time was a young man named Jeffrey Najarian. He has given me full permission to share his experiences here.

Jeff became, and remains, a TARA Approach Advanced Practitioner and Teacher. What happened to him when he began using the self-care that I taught him was clinically tested because he was HIV positive and under close medical supervision. Following is what he reported.

My T cells went from 77 to 520 with continued use of the TARA Approach. They doubled within two months of my first self-care class, and my daily application of the Main Central Vertical Flow [see figure 3.1, p. 27]. In addition, these applications completely reversed severe peripheral neuropathy in my feet. I also moved out of depression for the first time. I had struggled with depression for more than a decade, exploring every possible avenue of help, but this empowering application was amazingly different. I could treat myself for forty-five minutes and within that short space of time something amazing happened within me and I came away refreshed, revived, and positive.

What I aimed to evoke for the people living with HIV and AIDS who helped me develop the TARA Approach for them was the memory of who they truly are. I was mentoring them to know that they were not a diagnosis, just as I had learned that I was not my trauma. The imperative to make this discovery as death loomed added fuel to my growing understanding of the Rivers of Splendor and how and why they make the Art of Compassion distinct from other energy medicine systems. Even after the discovery of the protease inhibitors that, in the United States, lessened the death threat of AIDS, the quest for self-discovery never lost momentum for people like Jeff Najarian.

Something else that was completely momentous happened for me during the AIDS epidemic. That crisis gave me my first experience of healing in community. I was one in a cadre of health care professionals who rallied around the AIDS community and dared to defy the stigma associated with touching, holding the hands of—perhaps even embracing—and loving people with AIDS.

Through affiliation with organizations like ACT UP and AIDS Medicine and Miracles, I participated in, and sometimes organized, assemblies where healing was taught, grief ceremonies were enacted, losses were acknowledged, and communities were celebrated. I became part of a colorful, vibrant, and thoroughly creative tribe of outliers with nothing to lose. In our gatherings we sang, danced, recited poetry, screamed, cried, raged, and loved each other madly, unconditionally, and fearlessly. All of it was medicine.

My life as a survivor of domestic violence and sexual abuse had been cloaked in secrecy and shame. I was trained to disguise these wounds and to live with the fear they would be exposed. Now I was suddenly in groups of people who had been shamed for what happened to them and vilified for their suffering, and they were done apologizing for it. They were ready to declare their truth to the world. As I attended gathering after gathering, looking into the faces of people who were living a death sentence, who had lost their dearest friends, their family members, and who were memorializing their losses together, my personal shame was alchemized by the power of our connectedness. There is no shame in connectedness.

Because of Jeff and others like him I was motivated to continue the evolution of the TARA Approach. This voice of my embryonic being was needed and sorely wanted in the world. My ever ready and passionate curiosity, the essence of my embryonic self, was hot on the trail of psychoneuroimmunology, epigenetics, mind-body wholeness, and embryogenesis. Where did patterns of vulnerability originate? Why did some who were exposed to AIDS die from it while others were never infected? How did some respond well to the medicines while others were sickened by them? These driving questions, echoed within me, unrelentingly driving me to more research, inquiry, consultation, and formulation. The result was a simple protocol for remembering and claiming Original Brilliance. I call this the Rediscovery Journey.™

The Rediscovery Journey template decidedly points to several aspects of the paradigm shift in health care that I have come to espouse. This paradigm shift was seeded in many regards by my service during the AIDS epidemic. It is a potent message for the world's current crises, both climate and health care. The central aspects of the rediscovery process are what informs the attuned language of the TARA Approach. These aspects are:

1. The reclamation of our earliest, most formative, and influential developmental history in utero and during the primal period of life;
2. The unified field of consciousness that is the property of Embryonic Intelligence and is an undying birthright for every human being;
3. The integration of the parts of the self that have been fragmented at the causative level;
4. The identification of entelechy, or the seed of purpose, which is highly differentiated for each person and, once claimed, serves as a voice for our living Earth; and
5. The infusion of the will, motivation, and clarity to put entelechy into action.

While the resolution of shock and trauma defined my inquiries, research, studies, and the mentorship I sought from various teachers, looming behind this orientation was something beyond trauma and even beyond individual experiences of satisfaction, wholeness, and well-being. The AIDS epidemic introduced me to collective trauma and collective shock, and this led to the possibility of collective healing, which is dependent on the evolution of consciousness. In the service of that evolution, and to the principles named above as component parts of the paradigm shift in health care that I intend,

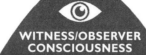

WITNESS/OBSERVER CONSCIOUSNESS

The highest consciousness, which is closest to God; compassionate, the detached, pure, and profoundly perceptive observer who sees below the surface of everything.

Sees and names true need(s).

THE REDISCOVERY JOURNEY™

THE THREE ASPECTS OF THE TRANSFORMATIONAL TRINITY

MATURE WISE ADULT

The part of consciousness that is parental, attuned, and not self-serving.

Answers true need(s) as well as committing to holding the child permanently in their consciousness.

THE CHILD OR PRENATE

The young self that has been wounded or has not completely met the milestone of some particular developmental need(s).

Receives and responds to the attunement, attachment, and bonding that is offered.

Figure 5.1. The components of the Rediscovery Journey

the Rediscovery Journey was born. The goal of promulgating it was so grand it sometimes frightened me. I heard the voices of all those who tried to forbid, silence, and squelch my embryonic vision. I dared to believe that consciousness could and would evolve to implement compassionate health care to everyone as a human birthright.

6

What Are the Rivers of Splendor?

In some ways you can think of these vessels like the Holy Grail.

YVONNE R. FARRELL

The Rivers of Splendor restore the core of being where shock strikes.

STEPHANIE MINES

Prenatal life is a university of sensory intelligence. It is the athletic field of evolving bio-identity. Each individual has a completely unique prenatal experience. Alongside the unfolding of organs, limbs, muscles, tendons, joints, and all the articulations of movement that build structure and function, there are energetic or bioelectrical accompaniments to action and being. The Rivers of Splendor are the channels or vessels that accompany embryogenesis. The Sacred Sites are the tributaries that flow into these rivers.

Bioelectrical forces weave matter and purpose—form and intention. They infuse each developmental cycle, from the very beginning of life, until its end. You—meaning your embryonic self—designs what acupuncturist Yvonne Farrell calls your "curriculum," or the physiology of your unfolding purpose. Bioelectrical and hormonal forces cohere into conduits that inform the flow of the Rivers of Splendor—a merger of genetic and epigenetic factors and the unique contribution you bring to that mix.

You have already met the central channel, the Main Central Vertical Flow (see figure 3.1 on page 27), or primary River of Splendor. She is the Master Weaver, the coordinating force that drives purpose into form. She embodies, restores, and ignites perfect alignment. She is the bioelectricity of your midline, which she can, if signaled, resuscitate each time it is damaged. Whenever we enact the ritual of this flow in any of its forms, we reinforce our memory of this birthright. The other conduits are her servants or her handmaidens. You will be introduced to them in these pages.

The Rivers of Splendor never cease being available to us. They may be burdened or suppressed, but we always have the capacity to relieve them of stressors. You revivify these channels through touch and awareness and thereby reignite your personal life force. This can happen at any age. You are never too old or too young to swim in the waters of the Rivers of Splendor. One of the purposes of this book is to reunite you with this birthright.

THE SACRED SITES AND
THE RIVERS OF SPLENDOR

The Sacred Sites are the recharging stations of the Rivers of Splendor. They are the power points for bio-identity. When I received this template, it marked a point of departure. It was a numinous, revelatory moment, though I could not acknowledge it at the time. It was, and it continues to be, a personalized experience of hope and companionship, meeting me as who I am with every touch. Even from my first awkward engagement with the Sacred Sites, I did not sense they were outside of me. I recognized the meeting with myself in a way that I can now call sensory but was then simply mystery. From the standpoint of neuroscience, I was turning on latent expression that had been put in the off position by trauma, shock, colonialism, misogyny, and manipulative cultural distortions.

The Map of the Sacred Sites is a physiological, emotional, and spiritual ally to whomever befriends it. It meets all illnesses and injuries with relief and insight. It recalibrates nervous system function and thereby all responses to the world. It is always accessible, no matter what the circumstances. It is utterly reliable and dependable as a resource that one cannot lose. It is the best of all friends, with no possibility of loss, abandonment, or betrayal. No matter what the duration of self-care, resilience is always awakened.

I don't think I am the only person who was raised with virtually no orientation to my body or how to respect and regenerate it. Through the practices of the Art of Compassion, I was stunned to discover that my body is a resource and that I could interact with it, learn from it, and regenerate it and my entire being. The regeneration I refer to here is the particular function of the Rivers of Splendor. I have designed a map to share with you, based on what I received from Mary, along with one created specifically for children and another one for our four-legged companion friends (see pages 50–52). The Rivers of Splendor are constructed of these sites, held in different combinations, with the express purpose of reminding you, physiologically, of your Original Brilliance— your embryonic radiance.

The Rivers of Splendor are named:

- The Main Central Vertical Flow
- The Diagonal Mediator Flow
- The Supervisory Flows
- The Mother Flow (also known by its focus on Sacred Site #13)

- The Wash Your Heart with Laughter Flows (the Left 15 Flow and the Right 15 Flow, also known by their focus on Sacred Site #15)

Their energetic interaction is depicted in figure 6.1. Each of the Rivers of Splendor are vitalized through flow sequences that combine the Sacred Sites.

CLINICAL RESEARCH DOCUMENTS THE RIVERS OF SPLENDOR AS MICROSCOPIC CHANNELS

In the 1960s a Korean scientist named Bonghan Kim (also known as Kim Bonghan) discovered novel threadlike structures that were called, at various times, ducts or corpuscles. These ducts, microscopically detected, contain fluids that are highly responsive to stimulation. They express their responses through bioelectricity. While these ducts, vessels, or channels, are around acupuncture points, they are distinct from them. Dr. Bonghan Kim referred to their special capacities to signal functional shifts. Since then, various researchers have documented these channels and added language to describe them, such as cell membranes emitting cellular activity in the form of voltage. Studies conducted in 2013 investigated further and renamed the ducts Bonghan Channels (after Dr. Kim Bonghan) and posited that they contain DNA. These channels are also called the primo vascular system. Research is ongoing, and papers continue to be published in acupuncture journals and from research laboratories in South Korea, including at Kyung Hee University, the Korea Institute of Oriental Medicine, and Korea University. Sang Hyun Park Ph.D. is a primary investigator. Some of this ongoing microscopic and bioelectrical research has detected that these threadlike structures could potentially be considered a circulatory system and that this system develops in utero. It is posited by acupuncturists and OMDs (Oriental Medical Doctors) that these channels validate the Extraordinary Meridians, or Rivers of Splendor.

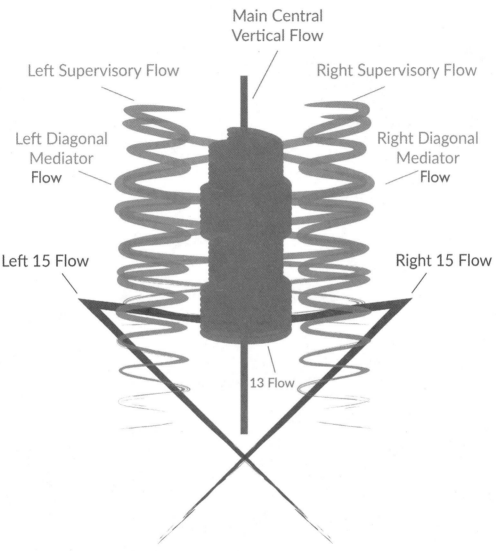

Figure 6.1. Rivers of Splendor diagram

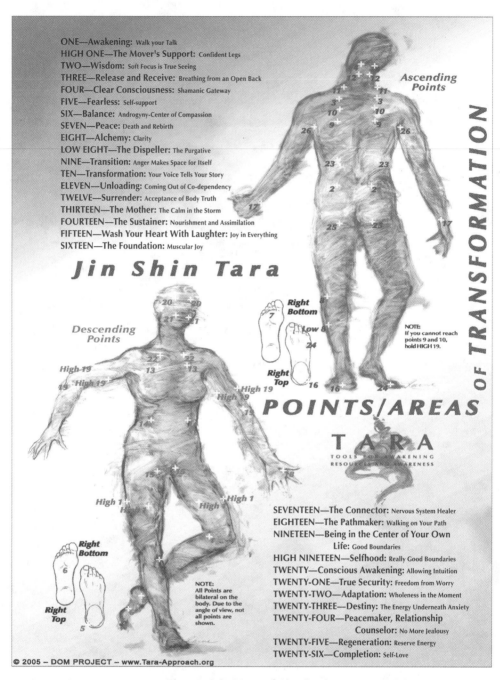

ONE—Awakening: Walk your Talk
HIGH ONE—The Mover's Support: Confident Legs
TWO—Wisdom: Soft Focus is True Seeing
THREE—Release and Receive: Breathing from an Open Back
FOUR—Clear Consciousness: Shamanic Gateway
FIVE—Fearless: Self-support
SIX—Balance: Androgyny-Center of Compassion
SEVEN—Peace: Death and Rebirth
EIGHT—Alchemy: Clarity
LOW EIGHT—The Dispeller: The Purgative
NINE—Transition: Anger Makes Space for Itself
TEN—Transformation: Your Voice Tells Your Story
ELEVEN—Unloading: Coming Out of Co-dependency
TWELVE—Surrender: Acceptance of Body Truth
THIRTEEN—The Mother: The Calm in the Storm
FOURTEEN—The Sustainer: Nourishment and Assimilation
FIFTEEN—Wash Your Heart With Laughter: Joy in Everything
SIXTEEN—The Foundation: Muscular Joy

Jin Shin Tara

Ascending Points

Descending Points

NOTE:
If you cannot reach points 9 and 10, hold HIGH 19.

Right Bottom
Low 8
Right Top

POINTS/AREAS

of TRANSFORMATION

TARA
TOOLS FOR AWAKENING
RESOURCES AND AWARENESS

NOTE:
All Points are bilateral on the body. Due to the angle of view, not all points are shown.

Right Bottom
Right Top

SEVENTEEN—The Connector: Nervous System Healer
EIGHTEEN—The Pathmaker: Walking on Your Path
NINETEEN—Being in the Center of Your Own
Life: Good Boundaries
HIGH NINETEEN—Selfhood: Really Good Boundaries
TWENTY—Conscious Awakening: Allowing Intuition
TWENTY-ONE—True Security: Freedom from Worry
TWENTY-TWO—Adaptation: Wholeness in the Moment
TWENTY-THREE—Destiny: The Energy Underneath Anxiety
TWENTY-FOUR—Peacemaker, Relationship
Counselor: No More Jealousy
TWENTY-FIVE—Regeneration: Reserve Energy
TWENTY-SIX—Completion: Self-Love

© 2005 – DOM PROJECT – www.Tara-Approach.org

Figure 6.2. Map of the body

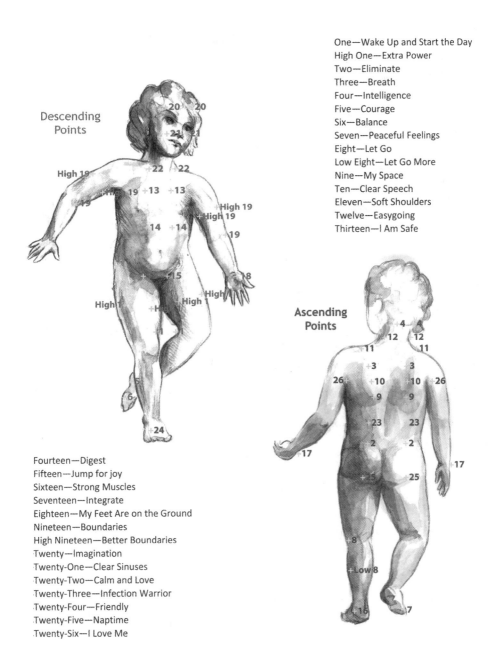

One—Wake Up and Start the Day
High One—Extra Power
Two—Eliminate
Three—Breath
Four—Intelligence
Five—Courage
Six—Balance
Seven—Peaceful Feelings
Eight—Let Go
Low Eight—Let Go More
Nine—My Space
Ten—Clear Speech
Eleven—Soft Shoulders
Twelve—Easygoing
Thirteen—I Am Safe

Descending
Points

Ascending
Points

Fourteen—Digest
Fifteen—Jump for joy
Sixteen—Strong Muscles
Seventeen—Integrate
Eighteen—My Feet Are on the Ground
Nineteen—Boundaries
High Nineteen—Better Boundaries
Twenty—Imagination
Twenty-One—Clear Sinuses
Twenty-Two—Calm and Love
Twenty-Three—Infection Warrior
Twenty-Four—Friendly
Twenty-Five—Naptime
Twenty-Six—I Love Me

Figure 6.3. Map of the child body

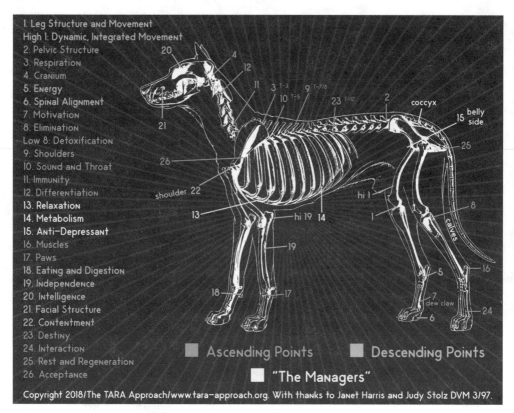

Figure 6.4. Map of the animal body

◆ ◆ ◆

The Rivers of Splendor serve hand in hand with the elements of nature. Indeed, they weave the symbiotic kinship between human development and the natural world. Mary referenced this reciprocity but did not provide the detail I have since drawn out, expanding on the skeleton templates she transmitted. What surprised me most as I was fleshing out Mary's references to the elements was that it evoked not only a new perspective on the resolution of shock and trauma. It also awakened a personal, psychic shift in the form of direct communication from the natural world.

The Rivers of Splendor and
Their Prenatal Functions*

The Main Central Vertical Flow (see figure 3.1 on page 27) provides a sense of wholeness and integrity. This flow maintains our connection to the Divine pre- and postnatally, sustaining a sense of inherent worth. The translation of this flow from the Japanese is "I am the Divine Presence in the Honorific Center of the Universe." This River emerges immediately upon conception and continues to evolve throughout life.

The Supervisory Flows allow the fetus to experience dynamic movement-based embodiment. These Rivers empower the limbs and extremities so they can reach, gesture, and make contact with the self and the environment in utero and postnatally. These Rivers are designed to allow the right and left sides of the body to have purpose, strength, and integrity of expression and function.

The Diagonal Mediator Flow coordinates movement from the right and left sides of the body and the right and left extremities (arms and legs) across the midline. This is the integration of all human activity, including expression and communication, whether in social engagement or in dance or other movement activities. This River is essential for balance, and this flow integrates the right and left hemispheres of the brain to support evolving intelligence. It paces and sequences learning.

The 13 Flow provides an integrating function for emotional, as well as physiological, process and change. As the fetus develops and differentiates (including sexual differentiation and differentiation from the mother), the 13 Flow sorts, prioritizes, and organizes sensations. It manages the organization and distribution of reproductive hormones.

*This content was first shared on the author's website in January 2008.

The 15 Flow sustains joy throughout pre- and postnatal life. It is the 15 Flow that directs joy in movement. When loss and grief overwhelm the sensations of joy, then the 15 Flow is hard-pressed to maintain its function. Because it originates prenatally, as do all these Rivers, it provides the basis for the connection between joy and movement, joy and action, and joy and expression.

7

Elemental Gateways and the Unified Field of Consciousness

No other word (besides uncanny) comes close to expressing the strangeness of what is unfolding around us. For these changes are not merely strange in the sense of being unknown or alien; their uncanniness lies precisely in the fact that in these encounters we recognize something we had turned away from: that is to say, the presence and proximity of nonhuman interlocutors.

AMITAV GHOSH

I was born in the Bronx, New York, and lived in a tenement building there, closed in for most of the year. Even when the weather allowed, the neighborhood was considered unsafe for a child to ever go outside alone, particularly a girl child. My cousin was murdered on those streets, and I was physically assaulted and sexually abused more than once. After my grandfather died when I was seven years old, there was no one left to accompany me, except occasionally my very distracted and often near-hysterical mother. When I could find a place to escape to, I chose libraries and schools. Though my ancestry was rooted in the soil of Eastern Europe, no one spoke of that land because of the grief associated with it. It is only my healing journey that brought me home to my true family in nature.

Mary gave me some clues about the natural world in her references to the Five Elements, but she did not emphasize this in her teachings, perhaps because she was always trying to adapt them to her largely white, middle-class, suburbanized audience. It was my passion to uncover the true path of healing for myself and others who had endured unbearable allostatic loads that led me to what continues as an ongoing awakening to the natural world and how the elements are alive within us. Since this awakening took seed in me it has bloomed continuously to become a capstone for my discovery of resilience.

The Art of Compassion, combined with experiential revelations about the unfolding cycles of prenatal life and neurodevelopment, unified me and brought me into wholeness in a way that gradually thinned the veils between me and the natural world. I understood the language of the birds. I felt a guiding bond with trees. Communion became a constant when I stepped into the ancient forest that is just outside my door in the Pacific Northwest. This is an ongoing, highly personalized, and solitary experience. I go into the forest on my own, in silence, to be with my family in the natural world. This is not about naming the kinds of trees or birds I encounter; it is about being with them. I know these intimate meetings are the essence of sanity, even though if I shared them with some people they might consider me delusional. As someone who felt alone in her blood family, I have discovered the ecstasy of being alone with my true family. I call this the Metallurgy of Grief. It is a hymn to the Wounded Healer.

The Metallurgy of Grief

The Absences.
I have grown strong from the absences.
No father to teach me about
Business plans or athletics;
No mother to soothe my
Losses in love or
Provide council about
Confidence and inherent beauty.
These absences make mysteries into oracles.
They chart inner locations that
Are mirrored by roadless paths into the unknown.
I am prepared for devastation.
I know how to make something from nothing.
Like the octopus that grows back severed limbs,
I know about regeneration.
We who have been absent of connection to
Life's root structures
Find what we thought we never had.
When we enter the forest anew every time we go there,
We are welcomed by our kinship with
Trees, rivers, mountains.
We find our names in bud growth and
Never aging conifers,
Our birthright relationship to
All that is.
We are resuscitated
When moss breathes into our bronchioles,
When Maidenhair Ferns fan the Primordial Fire of
voices of the Living Earth
That were muffled but never destroyed.

STEPHANIE MINES

GAIA'S HANDMAIDENS

The discovery of the birthright of unitive consciousness, paradoxically, often begins with the discovery of loss. Loss resolves when we awaken to its opposite—unity with Gaia. Indeed, the discovery of an indigenous inner personal strength and a will to live stands out as the centerpiece when early trauma and shock are resolved. Going beyond trauma is true fearlessness.

As Joanna Macy said recently to a woman expressing her fears about the climate crisis and the threat of extinction, "You have no fear now because you are alive. Whatever you feared is over. Trust. You are supported." The support Joanna was referencing is Gaia. To live the experience of that support is the complete resolution of shock and trauma and the essence of resilience. It uplifts consciousness beyond anything we thought possible.

I never would have anticipated that it would be the natural world that would take me beyond trauma. The interface between my personal evolution and the evolution of consciousness as a result of climate emergency is another among the unexpected gifts I have received on the path of the Wounded Healer. I feel as if I have been recruited by Gaia herself.

The first element that I learned about is called Primordial Fire. This element is everyone's inextinguishable flame of purpose. What Mary taught was that each of us carries within us an eternal flame that allows us to persevere and manifest despite any obstacle we encounter. I did not know there was an element in nature called Primordial Fire and that it also existed in human beings. How does this correlate with human development? What is the evidence of such an elemental experience in the human body? For me, the proof is in the fact that I was not destroyed by my mother's attempts to abort me. Nor was I destroyed by my various encounters with death in violent relationships and political protests.

The evidence of Primordial Fire is in the triumph of people who experienced torture, childhood abuse, sexual trauma, and domestic violence and yet bounce back from being flattened to become wonderful parents, caring partners, and advocates for marginalized and underrepresented peoples. I am repeatedly awed by the generosity of spirit that flowers in people who did not have experiences of healthy attachment and bonding but who nevertheless emerge as compassionate beings ready to be of service to humanity. That is the evidential data I collected in more than thirty-five years of bearing witness to the victory of the human spirit.

This is the spirit we carry because all of us, in a variety of ways, were met by Odyssean-like challenges on the path to embodiment and emergence from the bodies of our mothers. It was by recognizing this that I have come to see the story-behind-the-story of my conception, which I knew had been a rape.

As I stated at the beginning of this book, the capacity to differentiate begins with remembering and voicing one's truth. We are told that we cannot remember our early experiences. This is a falsehood. Claiming the truth behind that falsehood is my act of differentiation. Primordial Fire is the element of differentiation. Discerning consciousness feeds itself. Consciousness evolves beyond your wildest imagination as a result of claiming the power to differentiate, which is the essence of embryogenesis—the evolution of the embryo. For me, this was epitomized when I reconfigured the moment of my conception, which I knew had been a violent rape, and saw it, for the first time, from the perspective of my embryonic self, who chose embodiment.

Conception: The First Point

My mother was lost
That night, in an unfamiliar darkness.
She was adrift, gone from her moorings.
And my father too,
Had never conceived of me.
Yet I reached for them,
Slipping through the cracks in their consciousness,
Gliding in despite their ignorance.

In the time of turmoil, I brought my peace,
A specter of love for all humanity.
I shed my light upon them,
Entering their fluids with my passionate plunge to
intimacy,
Infiltrating their juices with my intent.
And so, I became here and now:
I ignited the Power of Being.

I illuminated the path
For a life of glorious truth.
I came in the name of the Essence
That inflames this path.
I came to clear the way
For a ceaseless progression of honesty,
A parade of the myriad forms of love.

My own clear destiny
Momentarily parted the seas of their confusion
So that I
Determined and direct,
Could move on.

STEPHANIE MINES

THE ORDER OF THE ORDER:
THE ELEMENTAL CREATION STORY

*The development of the embryo is the story of humanity. It
binds us to the universe by energy correspondences.*

MARY IINO BURMEISTER

The Order of the Order in terms of human development, as transmitted by Jiro Murai to Mary Iino Burmeister and from Mary to me, goes like this:

> We emerge into form in stages, first stirring out of unfathomable spaciousness, the time before time, an emptiness beyond anything we can conceive.

> From this place, we begin to take on density and substance, manifesting another state of vastness, but this secondary level of vastness is visible, like the sky.

> Out of the skylike state of perceivable emptiness, we consolidate ourselves one step further as we journey toward form to embody unique selfhood. We do this next by becoming light.

> Once we are in the form of light, we await the right time in which to densify further. This next stage is into an element that is called Primordial Fire. This is the soul fire of entelechy, or purpose, the form of individuated haecceity, or flame of expression. Primordial Fire is an eternal flame. It is undying soul purpose. This element assures the continuity of the lineage of intelligence and passionate determination out of which we descend, and thus it cannot be destroyed, though it can be hidden, distorted, suppressed, obfuscated, or put into shadow.

Primordial Fire is the bridge to the state of density that is significantly more palpable and perceivable. This is our first material form, the conceptus. Mary named this as the Wood Element, and it is the wood of the tree bark, the stable form of rootedness that makes us of the Earth by being planted there. The Wood Element is the source of muscular viability. It empowers the capacity to be visionary, and it is vision itself. It is the energetic force of forward movement, the power to push away and differentiate structurally, emotionally, psychologically, spiritually, in all regards. The Wood Element is problem-solving action. It is strategizing and manifesting. It is the power of vital force.

Wood morphs to Fire in this cosmology. The Fire Element builds our vascular system and the channels of circulation. It also is the light in our eyes, the blush of love, the arms and fingers that reach for connection. It is the element of the artist. The intimacy between Wood and Fire also reveals how the Art of Compassion links intelligence with creativity, the mind, and the heart. Indeed, they emerge from the same connective tissue. While Primordial Fire is the eternal flame of endless lineage transmission, the Fire Element is the spark of inspiration—the sun and the moon that rises and sets. These cycles request reverence.

The Fire Element educes the Earth Element. This is expansion into soma—flesh. Sinew forms on this courageous voyage from emptiness to being in relationship; it is a joining with the stuff of the Earth and all her creatures. It is touch, skin, feet, and all that gives us solidity and confidence in being, in going forth as self. This is the place where trust in being in a form is manifest. The Earth Element is the digestive aspect of being. I am paraphrasing acupuncturist extraordinaire Yvonne Farrell here: because digestion begins in the mouth, the Earth Element connection to the stomach channel means we can articulate clearly about what best nourishes us. As it forms prenatally, this element gives rise to the postnatal fluids created in the process of digestion. Farrell's statement elucidates the Earth Element's central role in nourishment and embodied existence.

Earth Element gives way to the Air Element as we make our descent into the body. As physical substance increases, so does vulnerability and sensitivity to the refined particles in the atmosphere. This is a global statement. Those fine particles, both pre- and postnatally, are everything from air pollutants to toxic, annihilating emotions that waft through the currents around us and are intimately woven into the functions of breath and assimilation. What if every inhalation of life is also an inhalation of poison, and how does discernment function in respiration and elimination? This is the purview of the Air Element. The boundary between joy and grief can be sliver thin. If what we inspire is tainted with threat and if each breath is an act of faith, the disappointment is, literally, consuming. We stand in danger of being consumed by grief in this colonized, extractive, and industrialized world, where even people are products to be sold and purchased.

Research demonstrates the correlation between respiration and behavior, especially social behavior. Nicole Westman's inquiries into the neurodevelopmental effects of air pollutants in 2017 showed a correlation between aggressive, even criminal behavior and exposure to pollutants (*Journal of Abnormal Psychology*). In the same year Ellen Webb and Julie Moon published research in the *Environmental Health Review* that shows how the inhalation of the chemicals that infiltrate the air from fracking create significant stress that moves from the respiratory channels and the blood to the brain, causing anxiety and even depression.

This supports my hypothesis that the Air Element is likely where so many people are trapped in their evolution, particularly now as grief from exponential losses, alongside proliferating airborne toxins, permeates everything, whether or not we are somatically aware of those. From the millions of deaths from COVID-19 to the thousands of species lost due to climate change, we are living in a world of grief. Mary called the Air Element "sticky" because of the phlegm and mucus that keeps us stuck to feelings we cannot move past. I am suggesting that unexpressed grief is gluing humanity to a step on the evolutionary ladder. I also propose that it's only transformational healing that can free us so the consciousness we need to go another step is available. We are blinded by our unshed tears.

In my qualitative research into secondary traumatization (*They Were Families: How War Comes Home*), focusing on veterans and their families, particularly their children, I detail how difficult it is, and indeed how daunting it has always been, for people to share their grief and pain with others. The pogrom memories and holocaust tales that my grandparents kept to themselves, the secrets of my father's abuses, my mother's inability to speak of her loneliness and rage to her children all created a thick environment, an unarticulated keening, that I absorbed both in utero and after birth. I identify the Air Element as my teacher. It mentored me to become a Metallurgist of Grief. By transforming this lineage of grief I inherited, I have uncovered the resilience that unglues this sticky element and allows the joy of connection, even when sharing grief, to arise. This is the destiny of Air Element healing, and it's what is needed right now.

The Air Element educes the Water Element in the creation story of the Art of Compassion. The Water Element mingles genetic and epigenetic lineage into the flow of immunity, perseverance, and longevity. The Art of Longevity (see figure 9.1 on pages 114–16) is another interpretation of the Art of Compassion Kanji. This element in its fullness and health backs us up with regenerative strength. When we honor the cycles of water we know how to rest. The way the classical Chinese medicine texts describe the Water Element utilizes the word *husband*. We husband or support our own energy by not violating the wisdom of appropriate action and withdrawal, retreating easily when necessary, and knowing the beauty of stillness. Thus, our joints shake free of trauma and shock and fulfill their mission of enhancing and easing movement, and our backs are free of burdens we do not assume. The Water Element is the secret of resilience, and self-care is the process of whispering that secret to oneself, over and over again.

We experience the waning of the Water Element in our last days of life in the body. From the diminution of the Water cycle, we move again to Primordial Fire to exit this plane to return to the vastness from which we arose.

THE REDISCOVERY JOURNEY AND
THE ORDER OF THE ORDER

Our people were a circle, until we were dispersed. Our people shared a language with which to thank the day, until they made us forget. But we didn't forget. Not quite.
ROBIN WALL KIMMERER

I call my template for reclaiming early memory the Rediscovery Journey because every aspect of it is like a voyage to the depths of who we are and how we are formed. Each time we embark on a journey of rediscovery and repair the torn fabric in the tapestry of our lives, we come back into the Order of the Order. What Mary meant by the Order of the Order was the balanced order of the interaction of the elements in human development. We reclaim that order through the healing that presents itself in the Rediscovery Journey. "Instead of living in the Order of the Order, we are living in the Order of the Disorder," Mary said. That was never truer than it is today.

The path of the Wounded Healer is to find a way to migrate from the Order of the Disorder to the Order of the Order within oneself and then to invite others into that process. Another statement Mary made matches this, which is, and I am paraphrasing here, that this entire energy medicine practice recalibrates biorhythms, and when those rhythms are in harmony with the natural world, we are renewed. We come to live as creatures of the Earth, in kinship with Gaia and all the elements. Given the magnitude of the climate crisis today, this means that the disturbances to Earth cycles are felt by us somatically. We experience what the Earth experiences. This increases our awareness of climate disruption along with the motivation to counter it.

The Rediscovery Journey is the language process—the script, you might say—for finding the holographic landmarks in each individual's formative experience, when disorder created a necessity to compensate to survive. Just as we have to repair the tears in the fabric of life for ourselves, so must we support that repair collectively. This is what is happening now in the movement to counter the climate crisis, social injustice, health inequities, racism, and all aspects of the disorder that we have allowed.

Mother

She shows me her face;
There, where the old growth hemlocks and alder
Tower and crowd closely to one another.
Her cheeks are plump with lanky and beaked moss.
She is full with smiling at the sight of me
Looking back at her.
It seems not so long ago
That I listened alone
To the sighing of the night,
The violence of the streets
And the loud emptiness of
Narrow passageways, and
Sat to meals of frightening food
In the chilling, ceaseless gray.
Now 77 years later I greet her at last,
Author of my cells.
"I am your Mother,"

She says simply.
Her soft voice carries easily across
The cold, rippling belly of her Sandy River
As the gold confetti of the season
Flowers the graveyard of her salmon.
Despite our mourning, we are overjoyed to be together,
Just as refugees wearing barbed wire crowns of thorns
Meet at the border crossing.
The dirge at the end of time plays in the mist,
Yet nothing can taint the Primordial Fire
Ignited by this reunion.
"I am your Mother," she whispers.
Her hot breath dries the blood on our faces
As we melt into one another.
Fatigue evaporates like sweat off a colicky infant.
Though hushed with love, her words are amplified
Through the vaporous megaphone of my body.
I join her in the fog draped hillsides of spikerush and
hydrilla,
Willow and rushes, and in the
Dense, ropey underbrush of pathways glutted with
mulching oak leaves.
The moisture oozes through my tissue
As she teaches me to melt into this immersion in trust.
"I am your Mother," she repeats,
"And this is the way to fight;
This is the way of action,
This is the way to meet the ignorance of others who do
not see me,
Who do not know that I am their Mother."
My eyes are closed and when I open them

I look again into the old-growth canopy,
Into what once was the mundane vista just on the other
side of the river,
Out my kitchen window,
Where I stand to wash the dishes.

STEPHANIE MINES

8

Regenerative Health for a Climate-Changing World

The Earth and all beings are always moving towards healing.

JOY HARJO

If I can't dance, it's not a revolution.

EMMA GOLDMAN

As a youngster I had an ongoing visualization, an interior story, you might say, complete with characters, dialogue, and action. It was my private, internalized, bedtime ritual. The central plot involved the dynamic between illness and health. Someone, usually me, was nearly at death's door and needed help. Physicians of all kinds would arrive, with miraculous abilities to dissolve suffering. What the illness was and how the healing unfolded was the action, and this changed from night to night. The healing could include incantations, ceremonies, potions, and whispered secrets. My pillows played roles along with the stars I could see outside my window. There was no one with whom to share this unfolding screenplay, and without critics, editors, or commentators, it proliferated itself with extravagant beauty and detail. Nothing was uttered so as not to draw attention to myself; all the activity was within me.

In this inner theater of my childhood, I was always readily healed of terror and anxiety. My lungs would ease their grief-laden hauntings so that I could sleep. With my vision directed inward, strabismus disappeared, along with loneliness. Who is to say I was not actually visited by kind, compassionate physicians from another dimension who, recognizing my embryonic being, were teaching me about Regenerative Health? I had within me, in my shadowy nighttime, an entire hospital for the afflicted with assured outcomes of well-being, calmness, integration, inspiration and, best of all, play. There was a stage in this clinic with delightful performances in which pillow animals, tree limb shadows, and star beings relieved suffering through song, dance, and stories.

What a remarkable embryo and child I was and still am. She is the one who found purpose and joy in meeting and lessening affliction. The characters in my visualized dramas modeled the art of attunement, deep listening, and prioritizing the lives of children. It is only recently that I recalled the clinic visions of my childhood and saw that they were precursors to what I consider to be my most significant legacy, the implementation of Regenerative Health for a Climate-Changing World. This is what I refer to at the beginning of this book when I say that I remembered my future when I remembered my embryonic existence.

My prenatal self knew I would eventually manifest, at exactly the right moment in time, what she, as a daughter of Gaia, perceived as the greatest need for humanity—a design for Regenerative Health. It is my premise that such oracular remembering is available to everyone. We can remember our future by reclaiming our Original Brilliance.

Regenerative Health for a Climate-Changing World is a systemic shift in our understanding of health and health care as well as how health care is delivered. It restores authority for health and vitality to the individual and to communities and families. It confidently stands on the foundation of the relational, compassionate health care that is everyone's birthright.

As Rupa Marya and Raj Patel say in their book *Inflamed: Deep Medicine and the Anatomy of Injustice:* "Studying the ways in which systems interact to create health or illness is the leading edge of a revolution in the understanding of medicine. The reductionist understanding of disease in singular terms, such as one gene encoding one faulty protein or one drug targeting one receptor, can get us only so far. We evolved as systems within systems: There is nothing singular about us."

I developed Regenerative Health for a Climate-Changing World to meet this Code Red moment because I refuse to accept the death sentence proclaimed by corporations and political and government leaders. Instead, I listen to the voice of my oracular, prenatal self and remember my destiny.

I have spent my entire life preparing for this moment. I know we are biologically programmed for evolution. Despite evidence of an abdication of this physiological truth, I continue to have faith in humanity and its resilient potential.

I reference Uncle Angaangaq Angakkorsuaq of Greenland, who has been on a lifetime mission to melt the ice in the heart of man. He told us at the Climate Change and Consciousness conference I organized in 2019 that it was too late, and no one was coming.

Yes, it is too late, and no one is coming. This is the mantra I have lived with as a child, and here I am fighting for the future of humanity even after decades of it being too late and no one coming to meet the urgency of our climate crisis. It is because of my own life and what I have seen that leads me to the conclusion that trauma survivors are some of our best, first responders. Our lives have prepared us for these times when it is too late, and no one is coming. Our accumulated wisdom is now of the highest value. We are the optimum practitioners of Regenerative Health for a Climate-Changing World.

I stand with others like Rebecca Solnit, whose book *A Paradise Built in Hell* speaks to why and how we can trust a groundswell to prioritize the physical and mental health of our families and our communities. I have seen this over and over in my service to the families of veterans and the families of neurodiverse children.

I know what it means to fight with nothing. That is exactly how I have survived. And that is the wisdom that will stand me, and all other trauma survivors, in good stead as we build this groundswell to meet accelerating climate disruption. In many regards I have written this book to mobilize this awareness and to finally realize the dream of my young self through Regenerative Health for a Climate-Changing World.

When hidden populations step forward—like the *parteras* and *curanderas* of Puerto Rico when Hurricane Maria struck and no one came to help their people—we mobilize the powers of regeneration despite the data. That is the mystery we invoke.

I am committed to a vision of Regenerative Health for a Climate-Changing World that is within reach. This is my response to the failure of so-called leaders, the powers that were. We can do this by becoming Regenerative Health practitioners ourselves.

We are meant to meet this threat with the innovative intelligence that is innate in our nervous systems. We are, in this very moment, moving beyond trauma, even while it seems we are in the thick of it. We are, as a collective, breaking through to the wholeness of connection with the wisdom of the Earth. We are doing this at the grassroots level. That is what gives me hope.

REGENERATIVE HEALING STORIES

One must banish oneself from an empire of institutionalized medicine built on injustice and build a

better way of healing, along with others committed to the
same vision.

RUPA MARYA AND RAJ PATEL

Real-life stories of Regenerative Health in action in families and communities go unreported even though they surpass in value and drama what media reports and films portray. No movie star romance, no prince or princess anywhere in the world has a story greater in beauty and significance than the stories of how people, with their own hands, voices, and intelligence, turn affliction, pain, and suffering upside down. These breakthroughs to wholeness do not discount the benefits of medical technology for critical care. They do, however, frequently make that technology unnecessary.

Though governments systemically betray and dumb down human potential, humans defy that manipulation, particularly when faced with health challenges. Those with the courage to look within rather than be pulled out of themselves discover what humanized medicine means. As Angela Davis says, "Decolonizing is training our gaze on the origins of suffering and grasping it at the root." That is what Regenerative Health is designed to do.

What does all this have to do with embryogenesis and the secret of resilience? Everything. Read on as I draw the correlations.

HEALING IN COMMUNITY

The art of telling and listening to our stories reinforces our
humanity.

FUIFUILUPE NIUMEITOLU

The oral tradition has always been the central medium
for the transmission of human culture and knowledge. To
bring back storytelling as a form of essential knowledge is
in itself a deep medicine.

RUPA MARYA AND RAJ PATEL

Seeing in the dark, the evolution of sight, is initiated before the end of the first month in utero. It is the most complex sensory system to develop, and its evolution is part of literally every stage of embryogenesis. However, it is keenly operative in the first trimester, and, like the tactile, olfactory, and auditory systems, its primary function is to send locating information to the brain. In coordination with the tactile system, the visual system works to establish identity and security in the environment. The baby orients according to where the mother is focusing her attention, or where she is not focusing her attention. The baby follows the mother's experience very closely for both learning and survival.

The progression of sensory processing in utero is the key to how we remember, and remembering is how we differentiate sufficiently to claim unprecedented leadership and empowered selfhood. We are all meant to be leaders. The stories that follow show this progression and reclamation in action. The stories are true, but names and circumstances have been altered and multiple case studies are merged for the protection of confidentiality.

I have the great blessing of witnessing human transformation. I participate in the lives of people who feel challenged, threatened, confused to the point of complete disorientation, hopeless and destitute, bombarded and demoralized by overwhelming events and experiences. My observations and my own journey teach me that the innate capacity for resilience can be thwarted, but it cannot be destroyed. It is with enormous respect for the individuals who entrusted their stories to me that I share them here.

REFUGIA

Refugia's parents had done everything they could to Americanize her. While they did not erase their immigrant origins, nor feel shame for them, they nevertheless were intent on blending in, being accepted, and succeeding on American terms. Rosalinda and Oscar had already made significant progress in realizing their dream. They were proud and protective of it.

Refugia, their eldest, had an unquenchable passion for social justice. By the time she entered college Refugia's social circle consisted entirely of avant-garde artists and left-leaning activists. Instead of turning her stunning intelligence into something that would bring practical, financial success, as well as stability and security as her parents modeled, Refugia did the opposite. She took on causes that put her future—even her life— at risk. She participated in demonstrations, wrote inflammatory articles, and protested against the school that had given her a full scholarship. Her mother worried constantly about where this would lead, and her father's attempts to reason with her fell on deaf ears. Her brothers and sisters followed their parents' lead and enjoyed merging with American middle-class culture. Refugia felt estranged from them. Nevertheless, this family stuck together, and everyone clearly loved one another.

Southern California, where they lived, and the Los Angeles environs, where they now had their home, was a burgeoning, sprawling microcosm of the vibrant diversity that makes the United States a scintillating, unpredictable, and increasingly multiracial, multiethnic melting pot. Refugia celebrated her Latino voice and emphasized her cultural affiliation as strongly as her family muted it.

At her university, which teetered on the edge of Los Angeles, Refugia was known to see her studies through her cultural lens and to challenge those who were not inclusive. She was part of a clandestine student group dedicated to challenging the status quo regarding accessibility and privilege. They met in parks where Latinos gathered in all seasons, relishing the mild temperatures, the scent of jacaranda, the shade of the evergreens, and paths lined with stonecrop succulents. Sometimes surrounded by entire families barbequing a meal and elders dressed as they would in their native villages, the group plotted their uprisings.

Refugia fell in love with the most extreme, most rabid of all the activists she knew. Her intense commitment to inclusivity and outrage at injustice was now fused with another passion, one so strong that it blurred the lines between who she was and another person whose being seemed to consume her. Sometimes she felt almost possessed as she allowed her lover's vision to overtake her own.

Ultimately this led Refugia to betray her own values. She was on the brink of engaging in violence. At her lover's behest Refugia worked to fulfill a plan that gave her a sinking feeling in her stomach and headaches so severe she felt as if her brain had split in two. Even in her most outraged state she had never considered violence. At the last minute, Refugia backed out of her role in the plan. Suddenly the very people she felt the most aligned with in life were infuriated with her. They wanted to eradicate her because of what she knew and what they felt she had betrayed. They stalked and threatened her. They chased her down and haunted her wherever she went. They cornered her, beat her, and threatened her with worse. No one came to her defense, not even her lover. He was now one of her assailants. Alienated from her family, her lover, and her friends, Refugia was forced to go underground.

At the point of desperation, fearing for her life, in a constant state of anxiety and confusion, somehow Refugia rallied a faith she did not know she had. From somewhere within that she could not name, there arose a commitment to her own life, an indefatigable intention to survive and not succumb to these horrific losses.

She disappeared. She went to another town in another state and took a time-out from the school semester. She lived in secret for months, and after the initial shock at the turn her life had taken, this underground time revealed itself as a strange, isolated sanctuary. She had the sudden luxury of time and space. First there was the grieving, days and days of sobbing for what she had lost, and especially for the relationship with her lover. She had felt him to be her soul mate, her twin, her lodestar. She had leaned in to him with the freshness of first love, drifting in to the soil of his strong body as if resting for the first time.

Hope for a different kind of future emerged, seemingly out of nowhere. It displaced the visions she had of the renegade life she would share with her lover and her friends, a life outside what she had come to think of as "the system." This vision had to do with herself and what she wanted to do with her life and her energy. Refugia had her own formulations about the world she had inherited and how education was delivered. Her time alone took on an almost joyful, seductive quality, much like an unfolding mystery.

Refugia was like a Jew hiding in Hitler's Europe at the very end of the war, with the certain knowledge that liberation was close at hand. She kept the blinds drawn and lived with a tiny, secret triumph, the vision of a future as tender and innocent as the sliver of light that came in through her door. This was entirely sensory and completely confusing. Therein lay the seduction. She had nowhere to go, so she simply had to be with it, day after day. Though she was distraught, and still deeply confused, her heart was opening, or at least that was how she understood the pain she felt there and the shortness of breath as her chest, of its own volition, tried to widen and stretch.

The most surprising thing that Refugia discovered in hiding was her love for the world. It was for this love that she had protested against society's injustices. Her protests were acts of love. When she first considered this, she was startled. Day after day Refugia tested this insight like a chemist testing a formula. And day after day her examination confirmed that it was true. The confirming sensations were surging, calming, and irresistible. They seeped into her belly like an IV drip, bringing nourishment that had to circulate, slowly, through all the organs of her body.

Finally, when Refugia got wind that the heated situation she had withdrawn from was canceled and the group that had tormented her was dispersed, she gradually returned to California. Refugia had maintained contact with her family, so they knew she was alive and well. She was received by them with love and relief. Refugia swore them to secrecy as she made plans to transfer schools and start her life anew. Her parents helped, and Refugia found herself in another town, restarting her life.

Despite the novel sensations and insights that had filled her underground days and weeks, Refugia was still rattled by panic attacks and ached for the lover she knew she could never see again. She recognized that his influence and domination over her was poisonous, but she could not shake her desire for him. Distraught at how close she had come to acting against her better judgment, Refugia began to wonder why she made these choices and how she could find a sense of self, a center, a purpose connected to who she was now. She was not sure she could even name who that was, but she was fiercely protective of that elusive being whose continuity she had claimed. In retrospect she realized how close she had come to being maimed, raped, or even killed. It was not that she suddenly felt remorse for not following the instructions of her parents; she knew that was not her path. She also knew that her passion for social justice was still her heart's true calling. But Refugia had lost sight of how to follow that passion.

Restless, riddled with flashbacks, insomnia, fear, and often almost catatonic with grief and self-castigation, she was without a direction. Refugia could feel that she was in a dangerous place internally. She had lost weight, and there were dark circles under her eyes all the time. She kept up her schoolwork, but it was a struggle. She knew she had to risk telling her story. She needed friends. She needed a support system. Her dedication to continuity, though only an intermittent somatic surge of will, was her compass.

After some time of contemplation Refugia reached out to a women's group that a classmate mentioned and was invited to be part of a women's circle. Something inside Refugia had awakened to a way of discerning what was right for her. Through the process of going underground and then emerging from hiding, she learned to track her senses and how they oriented her. *Tracking* was exactly the right word. She had become a tracker for herself.

One of the members of the women's group Refugia joined was a graduate student doing research into epigenetics. She asked the others if they would be willing to be part of a study she was developing about prenatal exposures to trauma and whether these carried on to influence genetic expression, behavior, and physiology. All they had to do was complete some questionnaires and discuss them. This was preliminary to the actual research study, but it would help sort out some questions she had about study design. Were they interested? Most of them were, so they decided to proceed. It seemed like a good place to explore. It could generate discussions about their mothers and their relationships with them, which all the women wanted to talk about.

Refugia had actually hoped to avoid the subject of her mother, but she was taking a back seat while she sorted herself out, so she went along. She filled out the questionnaires and then engaged in the conversations about them, with the neuroscientist facilitating and documenting. Responding to the questions stirred everyone's memories of growing up. These memories became ubiquitous, even seeping in to their dreams. Many spoke about how their early lives were dominated by their mothers, because their fathers, for the most part, were unavailable. It was during these conversations that Refugia had flashes of herself as a lonely, frightened child.

She could not recall playing with her mom or being close to her physically, or in any way. There was a gnawing ache of grief each time she focused on her early years. She did not know what to make of this. Her mother was such a strong, supportive presence in their family. She was always ready to help, to prepare a meal when someone was hungry, ready to run an errand, find something that was missing, or whatever her family needed. Yet Refugia could not arouse a single memory of having fun with her mother as a child. She was mystified. Some of the questions on the questionnaire were about her infancy, and because Refugia had no memory of that early time, and when she realized she had not ever seen many photos of herself as a baby or even as a small child, she called her mother.

The first thing that happened when Refugia asked about whether she was a calm or a colicky baby, if she was breastfed, and things like that, was that her mother became offended. Why did Refugia need to know these things? Her mother launched into a lecture saying that what Refugia should be doing now is getting strong, focusing on her studies, and letting go of the past, not dredging through it. "What you need to do, *mi hija,*" she declared, reverting to Spanish in her emotional agitation, "is consider what lies ahead, not what is in the past."

Refugia was persistent, and after a while her mom relented and started talking about what was happening when she became pregnant with her. She spoke first about meeting Oscar. This was not long after she came to the United States and was living with a family who, for all intents and purposes, were strangers to her. Oscar was not only from the same country, he was from the same region as Rosalinda, Refugia's mother. They shared a dialect. Oscar was absolutely intent on stability and prosperity in the United States. Rosalinda looked to him adoringly; he was a savior for her. She thanked God every day for bringing him to her. The acceptance and the protection she experienced with Oscar was the answer to a prayer Rosalinda had not even dared to utter. When they married, in a simple courtroom ceremony, Rosalinda experienced it almost as a cleansing. It was a new beginning for her.

Refugia's maternal grandmother lived in a remote area in Latin America, on a finca, or farm. Conditions there were very hard. When the young woman who would become Refugia's mother left, she knew there was probably no going back. This loss echoed behind everything during her first days in the United States. She was flooded by recollections of her life on the finca and of her mother. Rosalinda was able to push aside this sadness and guilt when she was with her husband and when she was working toward their shared goals. Meeting him seemed to make everything all right. But when she became pregnant, Rosalinda felt helpless to fight against the flood of darkness that engulfed her but that she somehow managed to keep completely secret.

Her remorse was like a dark curtain pulled over what should have been a happy time. Rosalinda and Oscar were working multiple jobs. They had not intended to get pregnant at that time. They would have preferred to wait until after they were more settled and financially secure. Nevertheless, there was no question they would continue with the pregnancy. Oscar was ecstatic about the pregnancy, but because of how devoted he was to his wife and to his vision of creating a stable home for their family, he was also preoccupied with making a decent income. Rosalinda did not want to trouble him with her difficult feelings. She became artful at hiding them.

Hearing this story from her mother was revelatory for Refugia. She was trying to take it all in. She listened intently, tracking her feelings through her sensations as she had become accustomed to now since her time underground and not wanting to interrupt her mother, who had never spoken like this before. Refugia felt almost as if she were in shock as she listened, and she wondered if her mother wasn't also in shock because she looked so distant, so removed from the present moment—as if in a reverie. Refugia tracked both herself and her mother. She was intent on this utterly new experience of mutual transparency and authenticity they were sharing.

When Refugia's mother began to speak about the labor and delivery of her daughter, she disappeared even more into reverie. She shifted from English to Spanish and then, when she caught herself, apologized and went back to English, but then lapsed into Spanish again, without seeming to know she was doing so. She described how frightening it was for her to go for exams and visits with the doctors and nurses. She was not prepared to be so exposed among people who did not speak her language and were not members of her family. She had always thought she would deliver her children on the finca, with her grandmother and her mother present. She never imagined she would spread her legs in front of strangers and be strapped down and restricted—like a criminal.

As Rosalinda continued to tell the story of Refugia's birth her dreamlike state deepened even more. Watching her, Refugia suddenly saw, for the first time, that she and her mother looked remarkably similar. Their dark curly hair was tousled and uncontrollable in the same ways, though Rosalinda had made an effort to tie hers back and was showing signs of gray at her temples. The curls escaped and framed her heart-shaped face, which mirrored the shape of her daughter's. Refugia was enraptured—stunned at their resemblance. The depth of feeling that was coming through her mother resonated with her passionate daughter. Perhaps this was the resemblance? They were passionate women.

The birth itself was uncomplicated, her mother reported, even easy. That was a relief for her as she couldn't wait to get out of the hospital, where everything felt strange. At the same time, Rosalinda was nervous about being alone with her baby. She knew her husband's schedule would limit his capacity to help her, and now she couldn't work, so his jobs had to be prioritized.

After Refugia was born her mother's sadness not only continued, it wosened. Rosalinda longed for her own mother to be with her. Oscar was even more consumed with earning money and learning English now that he had a family to support. As his wife slipped into her postpartum depression, his determination to make a home as soon as possible intensified. He saw that as his singular purpose. He was on a mission. And he was succeeding. He was doing well and progressing. His English was evolving rapidly, and he was well liked everywhere. This was what he had worked to achieve. Oscar was determined to keep this progress in motion. It was his love language.

Confusion, guilt, and grief were a constant, even as Rosalinda tried to tend to her baby girl. Sometimes she resented that this child had come forward at such an inopportune time. She reflected on the way the birth of her daughter robbed her of the special time she used to spend with her husband, after he returned from work. Those times were almost completely gone under these new circumstances. Rosalinda never failed to care for her baby; she dutifully responded to every cry and expression of need, doing what she remembered seeing her mother and grandmother do with other babies, or what her aunties had shown her when they had children. But her heart was not in it. Her heart felt strangely, oddly, irrationally broken.

It was when Refugia was almost three years old that things changed. Her *tia* Felicitas, her mother's youngest sister, came to the United States and moved in with them. Felicitas took over caring for Refugia, and Refugia's mother was able to go back to work. At the same time, Refugia's father made a breakthrough and got a really good job. That was the beginning of the turnaround for Refugia's family. After that, conditions steadily improved. Refugia's mother became pregnant again, and her father's job status continued to upgrade. The time of sadness was pushed into a corner, like a forgotten relationship. Rosalinda erased it completely, or at least she thought she had. She had not thought about it at all in recent times, until the phone call from her daughter. For Rosalinda, it was as if it never happened until Refugia reminded her that it had.

After the birth of Aurora, Refugia's sister, her parents became U. S. citizens. Her father's earning capacity doubled. Her mother and father now spoke English as the primary language at home. It was rare for Spanish to come into their conversations, and when it did, it was only a word or a phrase. Refugia's father had a management position, and her mother had no need to be a cleaner at the hotels to make ends meet. Rosalinda was awash in ongoing waves of relief, almost pinching herself to believe it was true. She was free to indulge herself with fixing up her home and caring for her children without financial pressure. She felt blessed. Because she had kept that earlier time a secret, she assumed no one knew about it, and Rosalinda decided she would not know about it either. She was only sharing it now because her daughter asked, and Rosalinda felt she had to confess.

As Refugia gathered in what her mother revealed about her early years, she was taken aback. The mental list that she still kept, enumerating the activist code of detachment from personal needs, railing against capitalism and colonialism, and minimizing personal emotion other than anger, outrage, and accusation, insinuated itself. Yet she could not escape the somatic surges that told her with an inescapable sense of truth that she had come upon a treasure about herself. This treasure illuminated why she had made the choices that brought her to this place in her life. It began to dawn on her that she gave herself to her lover with such abandon, and to the causes they served, even at the risk of her own life, because she needed to do just that—to lose herself in someone, or in a cause, because she did not have solid selfhood. Refugia had learned that much from her general psychology courses. She knew the meaning of phrases like "secure bonding and attachment," and she realized she did not have that. Maybe that was why she did everything she could to attach elsewhere rather than at home.

Refugia knew that until she unraveled herself from the story her mother revealed about what had shaped her development, her nervous system, and her behavior, she would not know who she really was and what she really wanted. Her commitment to activism, to social change and everything that entailed, was unwavering. At the same time, she knew, quite suddenly and thoroughly, that it was essential for her to create the space to clarify her motives. What was most stunning was that Refugia knew this was the time to do this, and she had every right to seize it for that purpose. There was no question about this. Refugia let out a deep sigh upon this realization. Instead of feeling she had messed up, failed, and gotten herself into deep trouble, she felt that she was in the right place at the right time, awkward and uncomfortable as that place was.

Refugia was surprised a few days later when she received a phone call from her mother asking for another round of conversations about the questionnaire. She had not yet fully digested everything her mother had shared, and now her mother was indicating there might be more. This was unprecedented.

After Refugia's first questionnaire visit, Rosalinda found herself remembering her own youthful life. The early years of working alongside her husband on the finca to build safety, respectability, opportunity, and educational options for her family had become inaccessible to her. Her mother and grandmother were dead now. Family members, like Felicitas, who had managed to come to the United States, had built new lives. Felicitas had a career and a family. She was a modern, American woman now. They did not have the time to reminisce about that lush, earthy, and achingly difficult, often life-threatening, environment that spawned them.

Yet in the wake of Refugia's questions, Rosalinda could not suppress something else that she had never shared with anyone. While Rosalinda behaved as if Refugia's rebelliousness was incomprehensible to her, in fact Rosalinda herself had been a rebellious, wild adolescent. Her strict father set very severe limits on what his irreverent, tempestuous, curly-haired daughter could do, particularly when her body began to develop and her beauty was evident to everyone. The young Rosalinda was defiant about her father's restrictions and expressed her rage by becoming promiscuous. This led to a conception that led to the arrangement of a complex abortion, overseen by her father's grandmother, who was a *partera* (midwife). This was why Rosalinda was sent away to live with another family—friends of friends, only distantly known to them. It was an exile. Her father was outraged. These arrangements were made at great sacrifice to Rosalinda's family, and her father continually reminded her of that. It was through the family that sheltered Rosalinda in the United States that she met Oscar and fell in love. He was her redemption from alienation, punishment, and isolation. She revered him.

Rosalinda knew she would have to share all this with her daughter. She did not understand why, but her intuition to do so was irrepressible. When Refugia heard the story, she cried with her mother. They embraced, and something happened that Refugia had never anticipated—they forgave each other for everything. They forgave each other for whatever had kept them from feeling the love they felt now that the truth was out.

This story does not end here. When Refugia reported all this to her group and to the neuroscience student (me), a new level of clarity emerged, a new dimension of consciousness about what had shaped her. Everything looked different, including the world around her.

The group decided to offer Refugia a meeting singularly devoted to all the permutations of what unfolded as a result of completing the questionnaire. Refugia was hesitant. There was a lot the group did not know about her, including her political activities, her time underground, and her relationship with the zealot leader with whom she still felt a bond, even after all her new understanding. There was an additional burning issue she had carried all her life: Why was she the only one in the family who unabashedly proclaimed her Latina origins and spoke Spanish? What was her family hiding? Why did they masquerade as white people? Could this group embrace this central theme that, from Refugia's perspective, was interwoven with all the others?

Emotions were flying everywhere. They seemed to ricochet off the walls in her bedroom, in her classrooms—even when she went to the bathroom. She felt like she was in an endless labyrinthian web of new discoveries, each of them a discrete, crystalline thread. In a strange, chaotic way, all of it was completely wonderful—a vital work of living art, swirling around and within her. Her world was exploding. Priorities shifted instantaneously. Resistance and assumptions evaporated before her eyes, shaping her movement and articulation. Life was, she reflected, completely out of control.

"So why not, then?" she thought to herself. "Why not go for it?" Refugia said yes to the circle of healing with the women's group and the neuroscientist whose hair was as wild as Refugia's and Rosalinda's. She said yes, knowing that she would be completely exposed. She might even be arrested if she disclosed everything. Still, she said yes. For right now, yes felt much better than no, and because she was learning to follow her body, she went with the yes.

Refugia told them everything, and no one threatened to report her. On the contrary, everyone in the group made a commitment, out loud, to honor Refugia's confidentiality. One of the women, an attorney, assured Refugia there was nothing for her to be concerned about as she had not done anything illegal and those with whom she once was affiliated had disbanded without taking action, so she could be at ease on that score. This caused Refugia to emit a deep, audible sigh of relief. She realized suddenly how she had traveled on a narrow strip of borderland between life and death.

Instead of expressing alarm, judgment, or criticism, the women as a collective had only one question: "How can we help keep you safe? How can we be your shield?" They told Refugia how much they respected her daring, her intelligence, her loyalty, her integrity, and her perseverance. Refugia had never before felt so valued.

The group as a whole was intrigued with how Rosalinda's early experiences of loss and rejection had shaped her daughter who was born years later in another country. Was this related to Rosalinda's abdication of her language and her traditions? And what about Oscar's story? How did this weave into the epigenetic inheritance that shaped Refugia and her siblings, albeit in different ways?

It would take years for all of this to unravel, but you can be assured that Refugia followed the threads and rewove the tapestry of her life and her activism. Now she could truly come out of hiding. The panic attacks, remorse, disorientation, and foggy thinking that were the marks of shock after her journey into the underground, resolved. She felt clearer than ever before as she reshaped her direction in life.

CORA

I was simply looking for some sense that women might have worth. And I found it there in the old stories of my own native land. I found it. Filled with images of women creating, women weaving the world into being.

SHARON BLACKIE

Connections are crucial to well-being.

SUZANNE SIMARD

This is the story of a young mother who assembled a community of her peers in a courageous decision to end the lineage of trauma and debilitating illness in her family so that she would not pass it on to her young daughter. She is a model of Regenerative Health, along with all those who volunteered to be part of her circle. Each one of the participants in this healing-in-community project listened deeply within to say yes to the circle of healing.

As young as she was, Cora knew that health is really about wholeness. Because she, along with the other women in her family, had a chronic autoimmune, inflammatory condition, she had been to many doctors. None of these physicians, or their staff, had ever deeply listened to what she had observed about herself and how her illness behaved and felt in her body. Cora was aware of when inflammation intensified and when it subsided. She was sensitive to every nuance of pain and how it changed and moved, and where it moved from and to. She was aware of patterns of relief and intensity, cycles that were particular to certain events or experiences. She longed to share these insights with someone. Yet no one else seemed interested. Or worse, they looked at her as if she were making it up.

Her mother, who had the same inflammatory condition, told her to not pay so much attention to the pain patterns. "You're making it worse," she said. "You have to learn to just live with it; ignore it. It's an affliction we share in our family. It's our lot in life." Her mother would say all this while she was talking and gardening, or cooking, or cleaning. She was demonstrating to Cora that the important thing was to not give in to the pain, to the swelling, to the pin pricks in her fingers and the aches. "Just keep going," her mother modeled. And it did make her mother happy to sew and knit things for the baby, even with her swollen fingers, and to bake pies and cakes that everyone raved about.

Cora knew she would have to do something herself if she was to find out more about her autoimmune condition. The medical professionals would not help her; if anything, they would dissuade her of her curiosity, just as they tried to cut off her questioning by limiting their conversations to bureaucratic forms and intakes. Cora was not going to settle for this kind of humiliating and infantilizing treatment. This was exactly what her family found so difficult about her. Cora took her own curiosity seriously. She was determined to find answers and not suppress, minimize, or be silent about her questions. "It won't get you anywhere," her mother and her aunts told her. "You're just stubborn," they said. Cora agreed.

In the small town where Cora was born and lived, it was common for families to stick closely together and for the women to marry young and start having children as soon as possible. It also was not uncommon for the girls to be virtual replicas of their mothers. This meant not standing out, not speaking up, keeping family secrets, and certainly never revealing much of anything to anyone outside the family. It also meant, if you were a woman, not being obvious, staying behind the scenes, being soft-spoken or not speaking at all if possible. The women chose, almost unanimously, not to seek higher education, unless it was to become either a teacher or a nurse. These women enjoyed their crafts and the art of keeping a clean and welcoming home just as their husbands relished their yard work and car maintenance. These tasks were fulfilling and unifying for them, and Cora enjoyed the beauty and simplicity of their lives with these dependable patterns. What she did not enjoy was the constriction, the limitation, and the imitation.

Cora followed the script in some ways. She married early and had her first child shortly after. She did not aspire to higher education. She wanted to focus on raising a family. That in no way prohibited her from being studious and inquisitive. She read and researched voraciously. She was a critical thinker. She was also, by nature, quiet and introspective. It was not her style to be aggressive. At the same time, she placed a very high value on transparency. When something needed to be said, she was ready to say it. The problem she often ran in to was that her cultural environment put tape over her mouth. She rebelled against this in her own quiet way.

Cora was passionate about her intention to allow her children, the daughter she had and the other children she felt certain she would have, to be whoever they felt drawn to becoming without the pressure to fit in. She knew the only way she could carve a path of freedom of expression for her children was by claiming it for herself. Cora felt strongly that the immune issues she struggled with were related to the ways in which her mother, her aunts, her grandmother, and her great-grandmother maintained a tradition of voicelessness. All of them had autoimmune issues, inflammatory conditions, asthma, and eczema, sometimes to debilitating extremes. Cora had all of these too. She researched the correlations between the immune system and health whenever and wherever she could.

Cora was friends with a student of mine who was enthusiastic about the perspective on development and health that I convey. I had written several books by this time, and Cora had read them. Through our mutual friend, Cora contacted me and expressed her vision of healing in community, with the participation of her friends and her husband. She had seen this possibility for herself just as I had experienced that need when I was quite little. How striking! I was moved by this similarity of vision and thus inspired to make my paradigm of Regenerative Health available for Cora in response to her request. We collaborated on the structure. This took a few weeks to orchestrate, but in the end, we assembled in a clinic and created the healing space with Cora at the center.

It was humbling for me to be chosen to share this with Cora and her friends. I felt honored to be selected for the role of facilitator. In all honesty, and I was quite open about this with Cora and her friends, I approached this as a research opportunity. I wanted to learn about the inflammatory condition that Cora sought to resolve and also about epigenetics. These questions had been vital points of interest for me for some time as I had documented in my writing. I also wanted to know about healing in the community as a route to empowered health care, particularly in an age when the health care system seemed irreparably broken. This all transpired before the COVID-19 pandemic, which emerged two years later.

Regenerative Health for a Climate-Changing World, a structure I developed, is inspired by the work of anthropologist Margaret Mead, who spoke to the relationship between the evolution of civilization and health care. It is also inspired by what occurred in the circle of healing that Cora orchestrated.

As a neuroscientist and an embryologist, I knew that each individual was an ecosystem of personal stories—genetic, epigenetic, and cultural forces, as well as their own singular entelechy. I also was clear that prenatal life was the most influential developmental cycle in terms

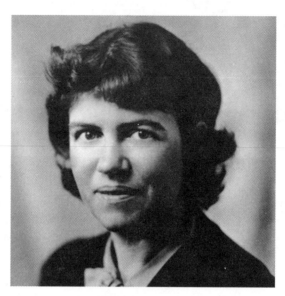

Figure 8.1. Anthropologist Margaret Mead, who spoke to the relationship between the evolution of civilization and health care

of establishing patterns of responses to the environment. Furthermore, I knew that health is never about one person but instead a reflection of all the interactions, relationships, and systems surrounding an individual. My priority was the nervous system as a tuning device, reflecting everything about an individual's ecology—the mycorrhizal associations, so to speak, of that individual and their growth.

Because Western medicine was disinterested, as Cora had noted, in the complex weave of each individual's health, I created an alternative structure. My focus was not at all on financial gain, paperwork, and industrializing processes—rather, it was on human beings, optimizing potential, and exploring avenues of well-being. I was informed by embryological research that demonstrated to me that resilience was innate and could be activated easily once whatever had blockaded it was dissolved or at least mitigated. The creation of a healing circle, populated by community members, was the best design, by my reasoning, to implement this possibility. A healing circle replicates the family sphere

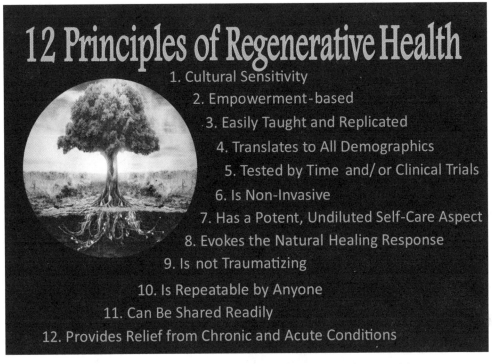

12 Principles of Regenerative Health

1. Cultural Sensitivity
2. Empowerment-based
3. Easily Taught and Replicated
4. Translates to All Demographics
5. Tested by Time and/or Clinical Trials
6. Is Non-Invasive
7. Has a Potent, Undiluted Self-Care Aspect
8. Evokes the Natural Healing Response
9. Is not Traumatizing
10. Is Repeatable by Anyone
11. Can Be Shared Readily
12. Provides Relief from Chronic and Acute Conditions

Figure 8.2. The twelve principles of Regenerative Health.

of influence. As such it has the potential to repattern responses by providing an alternate environment. While seen as visionary and idealistic by many, I was to discover later, in a pandemic world, that my design was not only of great value and necessary, but it is also rooted in tradition and has been tested to be sensible and effective.

Cora's Healing in Community

Cora selected all the healing circle participants and their roles. She identified the process that would allow her to be the most receptive. Inherent in the design is deep listening, and the person we were listening to the most deeply was Cora. What happens in the course of the process, however, is unpredictable. It is a qualitative research process for everyone. I am confident, based on my experience, that every single participant benefits deeply and is reflected in the process even though it is created by and for one individual. The reports from Cora's circle and others since is that this is correct. Following is how Cora's healing circle unfolded.

There were several musicians present, including Cora's husband, so this added the glorious dimensions of song and sound. Healing in community reflects the cultural elements that resonate with the individual at the center. For Cora, music helped her nervous system relax. She also wanted participants to speak up for themselves. Anything other than outspoken honesty was threatening to her, and always had been. Cora is petite, and her face cannot mask her feelings. She is without guile or pretense. Her bright eyes sparkle, and while you might think she is shy because of how soft-spoken she is, the vitality and strength of her being is evident to those who are sensitive and paying attention. Cora does not insert herself, but she is unquestionably engaged in all interactions and all the spaces she inhabits.

What is most distinctive about Cora is that she clearly has not lost the wonder of childhood. While her struggles with her family systems weighed heavily on her, along with her immune system difficulties and financial challenges, she remained open to the unexpected—curious and genuinely optimistic. Oddly, she suspected that this offended the other women in her family. She wondered why. Through the healing circle and the inquiries associated with it, we discovered that Cora embodied what the women in her family had forgotten about their lineage of powerful creativity and leadership.

There was a story the family would sometimes repeat from when Cora's mother was pregnant with her. They said her mom would spend hours at the graveyard, visiting the family burial site. Everyone thought that was really strange. No one, not even Cora's mother, understood it. She felt comfortable being near the graves of her ancestors, the people who had come to this country from Ireland and who had first farmed and raised cattle on the land where the family still lived. Little more was known about these elders, and the magnetism to the graveyard passed after Cora was born.

As we sat together to evolve a skeletal design for her gathering, Cora expressed that she felt something quite unusual was happening to her. She felt nourished as she reflected on the potential roles each of her friends and her husband would play. When she used the word *nourishment,* she told me, she meant that she felt like she was filling up—gaining substance and strength. She literally began to feel fed at a root or mycorrhizal level—as if she were receiving a serum of sorts that was repairing her where she was mysteriously, invisibly wounded. This was just from envisioning the healing circle!

Cora was bringing together friends who were not her blood kin but who felt like another family, a family of those who saw her and vouched for her unconditionally. These were the people who Cora felt recognized who she was. They were almost as curious as she was about her immune system. She had been speaking to them about her life for some time. They knew her well.

Was Cora's immune system genetically programmed to be weak, to react inappropriately and undermine rather than protect her? Or could she do something about this inherited pattern of self-sabotage? Was it possible to end this chronic pattern so her children would not replicate it? Was there anything emotional or psychological that made her so prone to inflammation? Was the held-back, restrained, even apparently suppressed quality of her mother's behavior that was the mirror image of her grandmother and her aunties related to this autoimmune pattern? These questions had plagued Cora for years.

Cora had explored the role of diet in regard to inflammation. She and her husband grew their own food and were very careful about everything they ate. She saw this helped, but it did not end the inflammatory flare-ups that afflicted her joints and sometimes kept her from being active and, more and more now, prevented her from holding her child in her arms for extended periods. She worried about this as she watched her daughter grow. She wanted to be able to keep up with her, but now she had periods when movement was difficult. During pregnancy and in the month following delivery, Cora felt liberated from the inflammatory pattern that had plagued her for her entire life. She thought she was done with it, but now, as her daughter was moving away from nursing and becoming more independent, the joint restrictions and pain were returning. This scared her and motivated her to inquire further.

What occurred to her now, in part because of how her intelligence and creativity were stimulated by envisioning and structuring the healing circle, was that there was a basic network of communication and connection that had been severed in her family. Was it the dislocation of that network that had produced this pattern of autoimmune dysfunction? Had the endocrine secretions of pregnancy and lactation acted as a kind of endocytosis or saprophytic stimulus? And was something similar occurring in the present moment as she absorbed the attention and care from a community of her choosing? Her questions were electrifying for both of us. As a result of our collaboration my entire concept of Regenerative Health was being enhanced.

Cora could feel, through her own deep, psychic attunement to herself in the supportive presence of people who were fully attentive, that there were storytellers and musicians in her lineage who had been forgotten, and many of them were women. What was behind this choice to forget? The only answer we could see was the colonizing and assimilative forces of the place they inhabited where unique cultural styles—like storytelling or musical vocations, for instance—were displaced out of necessity and more stoic and practical, almost puritanical lifestyles were preferred. In adapting and surviving, the storyteller, artist lineage was suppressed. With that came the shutting down of networks of vitality; the stunting of the polyvagal pathways that are toned by vocalizing, articulating, naming, and claiming.

In addition, the place where they lived was rural farmland that was regularly sprayed with pesticides, including the notorious Roundup that was praised by their neighbors because of its effectiveness. Cora and her husband refused to use Roundup on their land, knowing that it was a toxic carcinogen, but most others around them used it casually, constantly, and raved about the results and rejected other perspectives with vehemence. The winds inevitably carried the toxins to their land and infiltrated it, whether or not they chose to use Roundup. Roundup had colonized their families' immune systems for decades and was still doing so. It had also colonized and inflamed their minds.

There were many factors—genetic and epigenetic, environmental, economic, and social—that constellated around the perseverating autoimmune and inflammatory patterns of Cora's family. We considered all angles. Was it irresponsible to say the loss of storytelling, the cessation of the practices of passing down the artistic heritage of their line, assimilation into a dominant colonial culture that eradicated their uniqueness, creativity, and self-advocacy, could be causative for chronic immune conditions? This was one aspect of our explorations.

No one in our circle had any intention of disrespecting the health care providers whom Cora had seen and whom everyone in her family saw. The options were few and far between in their small town, so it was not as if they had a host of alternatives. Yet, this healing circle community trusted their own compassionate intelligence. Several people in the circle were health care providers. One participant was an herbalist, another was an osteopath, and another was a psychotherapist. As a collective we had confidence that our assessments and resources were beneficial and well informed. The structure of the circle provided a way for us to offer our views, individually and collectively.

Cora's circle concluded with identifying her and endorsing her fortitude and leadership. It took enormous perseverance for her to continue to honor her own insights when she was out on a limb by herself most of the time. We made a group commitment to back her up whenever she wanted to speak out. For everyone assembled, me included, there was the wholehearted agreement that our stories must be told to sustain our humanity and that silencing them was illness producing and inflammatory. Reclaiming our stories, particularly when those stories are about kinship with the land and impart belonging, frees the human spirit, along with the innate, vital forces of the immune system. This is not just philosophy, it is physiology. Research shows that speaking up—being vocal, rather than holding back, singing and expression—tones the polyvagal system and the vagal nerve in particular. This cranial nerve is the longest one in the body and unites digestion, heart function, and the brain. It may be a key to the anti-inflammatory aspect of the immune system.

The twelve cranial nerves differentiate and insert into the brain stem very early in utero—within the first few weeks. This suggests that patterns of suppression can be transmitted to an embryo who is acutely responsive to all the psychic and emotional conditions in their new environment. Before the end of the first month in utero, and continuing into the second month, the vagus nerve, along with the trigeminal, facial, and glossopharyngeal nerves, are differentiating from other tissue and innervating structures that become the throat, the face, and the internal muscles for the larynx. Thus, how the face reflects feeling is a product of the baby's response to forces from the world outside.

This is one of the reasons why, when we offered some applied touch remedies for the tension that Cora was feeling, we focused on releasing her face, which seemed frozen, with a deer-in-the headlight expression of startlement. Indeed, Cora reported feeling discomfort in her jaw and eyes.

Following is the energy medicine holding sequences we used to soften Cora's face, and it was recommended to her as self-care as well. We also offered her an incredibly simple but highly effective anti-inflammatory self-care option to continue to support herself.

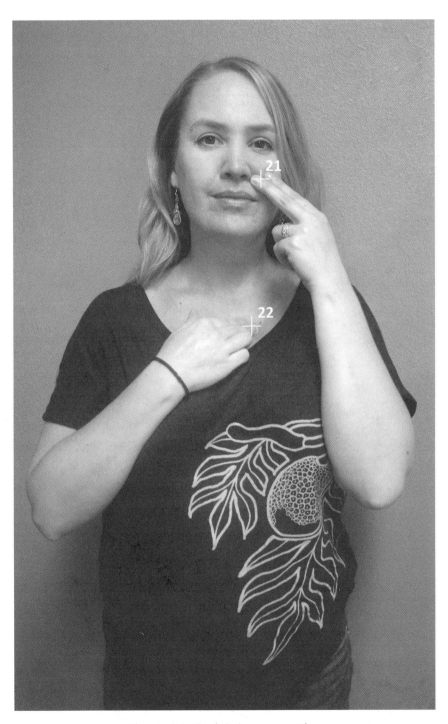

Figure 8.3. Facial decompression

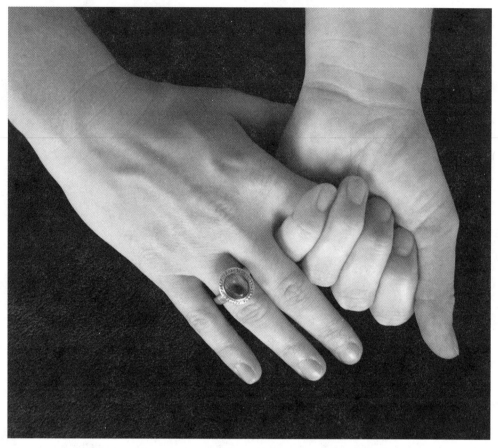

Figure 8.4. Anti-inflammatory application Inju

Cora stayed in contact with me after the Regenerative Health healing circle. She continued to learn more about self-care from me and with others. She gave birth to another child a year later, and the following year her aunt died of COVID-19. Cora stepped forward after her aunt's death to create an opportunity for her family members to express their grief. While they resisted at first, in the end the sense of loss was so enormous they needed to come together in a way that was safe. Wearing masks and sitting six feet apart, her family members allowed themselves to be led by Cora, who had learned from her own circle of healing how compassionate care in community is transformative, pain relieving, uplifting, and healthy.

PAUL

To find your mission in life is to discover the intersection between your heart's deep gladness and the world's deep hunger.

FREDERICK BUECHNER

The world desperately needs powerful storytellers to help us make sense of the unfathomable events taking place.

ALEXIS WRIGHT

Paul Craig was tormented. There was no other word that came close to describing his inner world. He was tortured by his thoughts, and he felt crucified by his loneliness. There were people around him who cared about him, but he did not have a way of communicating with them that relieved his torment. In fact, he knew with certainty that if he voiced his truth he would alarm and trouble his family.

He also could not connect with others his age where he lived. He watched as his peers, the very same people with whom he had gone to school and graduated alongside, found partners, jobs, careers, direction, and connection with others. He could not seem to manage any of that. How could he possibly articulate the magnitude of the confusion that raced through his mind and his body every day? He was certain if he revealed it that everyone would think he was insane. He himself wondered if he might be insane. He fought against the urge to confess his inner conflict to his parents because he did not want to burden them. At the same time, he was sensitive to how troubled they already were as they watched him withdraw more and more.

Paul was also sensitive to the tension between his mother and father. This weighed on him, and, like so many other things in his experience, he did not feel safe to share his perceptions with anyone else he knew.

He had learned, somehow, that he was dramatically different and that his differences brought with them shame. He could not risk being open about his awareness, his sensitivity to the unseen. He also had premonitions of what was going to happen. He felt that his mother and father would separate at some point even though they were a united front and cared deeply about their family. They never argued or were disagreeable. Paul wanted to ease the hidden tension between his parents, but instead he felt he made it worse just by virtue of being who he was.

After he graduated from high school, Paul decided to take a gap year. He got a job at a local bookstore. He intended to go to college, and he had a sense of direction about what he wanted to study. He loved literature, and he really wanted to write plays for the theater. He had already written a few. They came alive inside him and were his primary respite from the labyrinthian journeys he went on in secret, mostly with his eyes closed, while he sat on the sofa in the apartment he rented after he moved out of his family home. He could sit on that sofa for extraordinarily long periods of time. He became almost catatonic. When he did that at home it really worried his parents. His siblings just made fun of it.

Paul was a tall, gangly man, more than six feet in height. His dark hair was usually rather unkempt. He had to be reminded to tuck in his shirt or to brush away the crumbs that fell from eating his favorite delicacies like croissants filled with chocolate or crisp cheese sandwiches. He often seemed preoccupied, distracted by something, and thus inattentive to appearances. When he was engaged and interactive, though, he had the most astounding smile. If something intrigued, delighted, or pleased him and he smiled, even when he was tantalized by something like a work of art or a comment made by someone, his entire face lit up. This wrought a notable transformation, and others who saw it could not restrain themselves from smiling back. There was a marked contrast between his otherwise flat affect and withdrawal and his infectious smile.

This contrast was like the signpost at the entrance to the threshold on which Paul teetered. Internally he roiled with conflicting impulses. On the outside he was a pure enigma. Born with a male body and characteristics, Paul felt that he had a secret, internal sense of being feminine. He longed to present that way in the world sometimes, and that longing terrorized him. There was more. Paul felt the presence of other beings, and one in particular—someone with whom he felt deeply aligned, someone he knew was dead but was nevertheless in direct communication with him. No one he knew had ever spoken of anything like this. The only reading he had ever done about this led to a diagnosis of schizophrenia or criminal behavior. Did he need medication, or even hospitalization? He was afraid to ask if anyone else thought so, particularly his parents, whom he loved dearly but who were not well-off, and Paul knew that a path of mental illness could be costly.

At the same time, Paul was also full of joy. His own creativity delighted him and could bring that radiant smile forward. The creativity of others also delighted him, and nature was a source of ongoing near-ecstatic experience. The natural world was where he felt the most at home. He loved to wander in the lush hills outside of town or to walk the beaches as far away from everyone as possible. He scampered with the shorebirds and lay in the sand, soaking up the heat and feeling his connection to the tiny creatures, even the bothersome ants, who crawled beneath the surface of vision, making ripples that only an attentive observer could see.

What he experienced inside, though, was challenging to transmit into anything he could share with others. It took him hours sometimes to find the words that described his perceptions. Because of this there were long pauses in his responses to other people's questions, and that seemed to alarm them. Sometimes he wished he could be a musician, as sound came closest to translating his experiences, but he did not seem to have any ability with music. Ironically, words came easily to him when he was writing, and so that was one of his consuming interests.

Other than a few plays, he was hesitant about sharing his writing. So, his joy and his pain seemed always to be swirling together.

Paul contacted me after hearing me on a podcast in which I was enthusiastic about the arts as avenues of healing trauma. Because I am also a writer, and because I do not sugarcoat my difficulties, he felt he could speak to me about his struggles from the vantage point of wanting to someday publish his writing. He knew my work revolved primarily around health and trauma resolution, so he hoped our interaction would also lead to some new options. He felt proud of himself for finding me and reaching out without having to consult with anyone else, particularly his parents. He wanted to chart his own path, and he knew he was in trouble. Asking for help was not easy for him. It was always a risk. I recognized this almost immediately and felt he was a kindred spirit. I invited him to register for programs I was offering and to visit my website for books and articles that might speak to him.

Through classes, groups, and mentorship meetings, Paul and I developed a relationship that gave him enough safety to confess to me how much he thought about death. One train of thought that seemed to follow him everywhere was about how his death could alleviate not only his own struggles but also the suffering he felt he imposed on others, particularly his parents. They were always worried about him. If he did anything that they considered normal, like getting a job at the bookstore or renting an apartment, they were elated. They celebrated when one of his plays was chosen for an award and was performed in high school, but they did not understand the play. His mother, in particular, seemed disturbed about some of the characters and their sexuality.

Paul articulated to me that he felt he was not meant to live very long. His sense of disconnection, and of being lost in the confusion about his sexuality, never really resolved. The climate crisis was another reason Paul felt restless and unsettled all the time. He knew the chances of humanity surviving climate disaster were decreasing by the hour, and he understood why. People did not take the climate crisis seriously. Every time he saw someone violate the natural world he cherished, by throwing trash, carving their initials into trees, being wasteful and irreverent about resources, he felt more despair. He had no way to distance himself from this and, what was worse, he did not know what he could do about it. How could he make a difference when he was often almost unable to function because of his depression and despair? He had no way to filter out the horrific reality he inhabited, no way to protect himself from the onslaught of continuous bad news. Even worse—he felt responsible. If he could not act to make a difference, what purpose was there in being alive?

It was close to impossible for me to counter Paul's arguments about giving up. I saw the same behavior in the world that he did. I knew the future of humanity was in imminent danger. At the same time, I felt that voices like his—the voices of young people—were the very ones that needed to be heard and amplified. I believed in Paul. I had seen his brilliant creativity, and I witnessed his beaming smile that, from my standpoint, could only come from a radiant heart. I wanted to help Paul find a solid, respectful, and enduring relationship with himself that imparted value for who he was and what he embodied.

The online groups Paul joined never really met him where he was. His gender fluidity continued to trouble him. Groups that focused on gender did not match his needs either. He needed intellectual and inspirational artistic alliances. These were not easy to find where he lived and where his family was well known. They were in a seaside community with village centers scattered along the winding coastline. Everyone wanted to know everything about everyone else. Paul did not feel safe with this. As an artist he had to percolate ideas inside himself. This required not talking about what he was thinking, incubating and developing concepts and sharing them with only a select few who understood his creative process. He had not yet found those peers.

Paul was a prolific reader. No one in his family liked to read or talk about books. Paul still spent most of his free time alone. The person he talked to the most, besides me, was Mr. Smythe, the owner of the bookstore where he worked, and Mr Smythe was seventy years old! When I asked Paul if he felt lonely, he just stared at me. Loneliness was not even a concept for him because that was all he knew. He could not remember when it was different.

Though Paul had promised me, and signed a contract to this effect, that he would not harm himself, he was at a dangerously low point, and I felt concerned when I asked him these questions: "What is missing in your life? What stops you from loving your body and caring about yourself? What do you need that will allow you to feel whole?"

Paul's eyes widened, and he glanced away, gazing at a corner of the room for what seemed like an eternity. I noted the tension in my own body as I sat poised on the edge of my seat waiting for his response. I used the energy medicine I practice to let go and differentiate from his situation and any feelings of over-responsibility I had in regard to him. Thankfully this helped me ease into a place of trust and acceptance. In the spaciousness that Paul's silence created, I reflected on my own relationship to despair, death, and suicide and how tenuous life seemed these days, with extinction everywhere and loss a daily constant.

After a few minutes Paul turned his eyes to look at me. Then, much to my relief, he smiled. It was that wide, joyous smile that told me we were on the other side of the abyss.

"I need to find my tribe," he said, in his long-awaited reply. "I need to find more people like you and Mr. Smythe, but who are my age, and who want to read my writing and listen to my ideas. I need to shift my attention away from the people who do not get me. It is not that I need to feel loved," he continued. "I feel loved. I just don't feel valued."

While I knew that valuing himself was the goal, I also knew that valuing self needs to be modeled and mirrored and that someone as unique and sensitive as Paul would know when that was missing, even if others were loving. If instead what is modeled is conformity and acceptability and meeting standards of uniformity, then the response can be self-blame and self-rejection when one's goals are radically different from the norm. Paul felt trapped in a body and in behavior that did not meet external validation almost anywhere. How was he then to value himself?

Value has content and substance. Paul yearned to be valued for the very differences about him that confused so many others. For this reason, he hit the bull's-eye when he named his need. His value needed mirrors so that value could be reflected back to him until he owned it. This was likely a developmental need that began in utero and was still waiting to be met. My awareness of the psychic developmental needs of prenatal life aided me in comprehending Paul's breakthrough articulation and the differentiation between being valued and being loved.

The next milestone occurred when Paul shared with me his relationship with the dead. It was clear to me that Paul was not crazy when he spoke of communication with the dead. I told him so. It was my professional and personal assessment that Paul could retain a sense of stability while simultaneously perceiving other dimensions. It was, however, quite challenging in a world that had forgotten its own humanity. The inseparability of life and death is a topic for poets and philosophers, artists, and seers. I saw Paul as one of these. If he were mentally ill, then he would not be able to function as he did. His functionality, I was confident, would only become more socially engaged, more embodied, as he came to value his gifts. This could happen much more easily, as he proposed, when he was in the company of others like him. We both knew those people were out there and that he needed to find them.

These were not usual times that we inhabited. In fact, they were extraordinarily upsetting, and young people like Paul, with great gifts of sensitivity, were shouldering the allostatic load imposed by circumstances they did not create. As a health care provider, a humanist, and a scientist, I had a responsibility to incorporate the sociocultural context into my services and to recognize that the old story of health care was broken, useless, and even destructive now. I had to bring my creative intelligence and independent, informed awareness of neurodevelopment to bear if I was to be in attunement with Paul and others like him. I had to be courageous in my own way by defying the obsession with diagnostics and pharmaceuticals in my field and instead listen deeply, trusting my perceptions.

Paul and I probed whether or not the visitations from the dead he experienced were attempts from guardians trying to assist him. He thought they were because of the kindness he felt from them. On a somatic level, Paul felt these presences as a wall of support. He often experienced himself leaning in to them to find his ground. Where did they come from? Were they particular to his lineage, or universal?

Paul's parents were very private people, but Paul knew there had been losses in their families—some of them quite tragic. His mother had mentioned once or twice that she had a twin brother who died at birth. Paul understood that she did not want to explore this further. His father was alienated from his family for reasons no one explained, but Paul had heard indirectly that an uncle had committed suicide and that his grandfather was murdered by thieves. These losses were like missing pages from a manuscript. Maybe there were other pages that were unaccounted for?

I had to respect the entrenched parasympathetic orientation of Paul's family culture even if I did not understand it. Paul had incubated in that culture and done his best to accommodate it. This was a sign of his giftedness and sanity—that he adapted and compensated as best he could to survive under circumstances that were, from a mental health and attachment standpoint, not supportive of who he was. Paul had inhabited that culture from the moment he was conceived. It was in his skin, his hair, and his blood. I was not part of that culture, but I still had to respect it.

"Never sacrifice the value of your voice," was the sentence that resonated inside me in response to Paul's struggles in the world. I had to explore deeply within myself to see if this message was what he needed to hear out loud or the one I was to model for him. I did not seek to put Paul in the position of opposing his family or his culture. This culture was important to him, and while he acknowledged that he had to find his tribe and set a protective boundary for himself from those who could not perceive him, still, he did not want to sacrifice his established relationships. How could I support his differentiation without challenging his allegiances? These are the culturally sensitive questions one must ask to truly be of service to another. I considered, because of what I knew about the epigenetic forces on development, that the same conditions that restricted him now were also present in utero.

I also had to differentiate myself and my own history from Paul's process. While I did not come from a culture of parasympathetic dominance, I nevertheless did have a personal history in which my voice of truth was squelched. I had reclaimed my voice, for the most part, by this time. While I felt clear about my own resolution, I still had to be circumspect and not transfer or project what I discovered and knew onto Paul.

The COVID-19 pandemic took a toll on the inbred, small community where Paul lived. They learned the lesson, though, and people woke up and took measures to protect themselves. This led to an opening when infections stopped almost completely before new variants appeared. Paul took advantage of that opening to relocate and establish himself at a university that had a strong liberal arts program. His ethnic background gave him scholarships and other opportunities. From time to time, he sends me his poems and his photographs. Some of them follow here.

The Haunting

Ribbons of blood stretch beneath silent explosions of stars.
Nights of solitude and slow, slow dances of death bring me
Strange memories of bones turning to earth.
What secrets are tucked in caves down by the shimmering ocean mouth?
She stretches like the black, curvaceous seductress that I want to be,
Rippling with her dress of flecked gold.
I reach for her like an awkward child hoping she will swallow me,
Pull me down to where it is murky, turgid, and thick with teeming life.
"Please," I beg the ocean, "suck me into a language for which there is no translation."
"Let me become the articulator of what is lost."
She agrees, making me into an iridescent being
Who one day will flicker out of sight,
Like a poem.

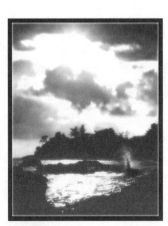

Figure 8.5. Wave splash.
Photograph by Tom McKinlay.

Sunset

They line up in the sky to honor the demise of the sun.
And then the warriors board a long boat and form
an entourage.
They chant through the night,
Songs of victory, songs of birth and death, songs of
the people.
The sky bleeds orange and turquoise tears for all
the losses
That float horizontally down to become palm fronds,
Lashes on the yearning eyes of tomorrow.

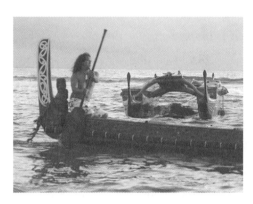

Figure 8.6. Traditional
Polynesian sailor.
Photograph by Tom McKinlay.

9
Your Resilient Embryogenesis

The embryo is our primary reality.

JAAP VAN DER WAL

E mbedded in the Art of Compassion is the energetic story of fold-ing and unfolding or embryogenesis. It is within this creation tale that we find the secret of resilience. It was when I decoded the Map of the Sacred Sites that Mary Iino Burmeister imparted to me and saw how it correlated with embryology that I understood the magnificence of the gift. That happened more than twenty-five years after I met her and when she was no longer available to teach or communicate. I had no choice but to unearth this secret on my own. There was no one to reveal it to me.

When Jiro Murai received the directives for self-treatment that saved his life, they seemed to come from out of nowhere. He simply found himself using the hand postures that are called *Inju* (see pages 114–16) and holding the Sacred Sites. What actually transpired, I know now, was that he reignited his essence; he restored the truth of his being. This is what he was always searching for. He found it within himself.

Jiro Murai turned away from his family's orientation to search for something he could call his own. He did not really know what that was, but he had to search for it, even though he frequently looked in all the wrong places, as so many of us do. While engaged in that quest he became so ill that he was forced to return to the very people he had rejected.

Through the ensuing process of going from a near-death experience to a kind of resurrection, Jiro Murai not only reclaimed his health, but he also reclaimed his birthright of connection to the world around him. He was awakened to a dedicated love for life and humanity. That is why the entire methodology is called the Art of Compassion. When I saw the correlation between the Sacred Sites and embryogenesis, I understood that Jiro Murai's discovery was not for him alone; it is a rite of passage for all humanity. I saw that the practice of the Art of Compassion would turn on the connectedness, kinship, and oneness that belongs to all of us. All of this must be found somatically because it is instilled in connective tissue. Philosophy, bullet points, and theorizing will not get you there. As a neuroscientist I was cognizant of the neurohormonal cascades in the process of embodiment and why the incorporation of consciousness, through embodied articulation, seals the awakening, manifests connection, and makes the entire process of reclamation efficient and enduring.

Fusing neuroscience, embryology, and energy medicine became my contribution to a healed future. I understand this to be the foundation of Regenerative Health, as well as my destiny. For Jiro Murai, it all began with the Inju, or hand postures.

Once the practice of Inju assured his continuity, Jiro Murai quested for the rest of the story. That took awhile to unravel. Even after Mary left Japan and was living in California, only a portion of the story was known. Before he died, though, Jiro Murai had revealed to Mary the entire Map of the Sacred Sites and how to use it to go beyond illness, trauma, and shock and breakthrough to wholeness. I translated that map into the story of energetic embryology, or energetic embryogenesis, as seen in the tables on pages 117–21.

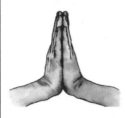

Inju, or mudra, derive from ancient, sacred wisdom. Repeat these hand postures as frequently as possible, maintaining focused concentration. All these positions may be done on either or both hands. The purpose of these gestures, according to their universal tradition, is to awaken you to your essence. They also have been known to reduce stress and fatigue, increase immune strength, and enhance vitality. Special thanks are humbly offered to Jiro Murai, Mary Iino Burmeister, and Haruki Kato for their transmission of this lineage which is our common birthright.

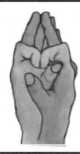

Great sun Diamond Inju
Index fingernails touch while middle, ring, and little finger palms touch and the thumbs also touch. Use this Inju to balance temperature disturbances such as extreme and unusual cold or heat when circumstances do not seem to merit it. This inju is a great help for circulation problems.

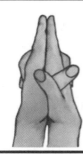

Kidney-Strengthening Inju
The palms of the index fingers touch while the other fingers fold together and intertwine, forming the image of a temple. This Inju strengthens the bones, balances kidney-adrenal function, enhances immune suppor and provides endurance and reliance. This is the physician's Inju.

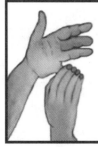

Outside the Earth Inju
Hold the inner seam of the little finger with the index, middle, and ring fingers of the opposite hand. This Inju opens the throat and helps speech flow clearly and easily.

Figure 9.1. Inju: The art of longevity (part one)

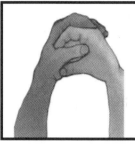

Solar Plexus Inju

The index finger of one hand rests in the valley between the index finger and thumb of the opposite hand. This Inju relaxes the shoulders, opens the solar plexus, and helps us to let go.

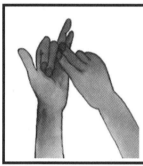

Heart Protector Inju

Hold the middle and index fingers down on the palm of the same hand. The middle and ring fingers of the opposite hand rest at the base of the little and ring fingers of the hand with the folded fingers. This Inju supports the pericardium or Heart Protector, thereby relieving the burden of multiple stressors.

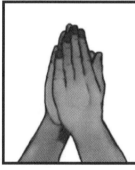

Palm or Prayer Inju

Bring together the palms of the hands and all the fingers as in prayer, pressing slightly to create contact. This Inju brings you into a centered place of presence, stops nausea and eliminates confusion, as well as provides focus.

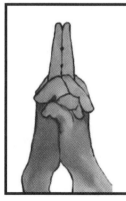

Fatigue-Releasing Inju #1

The palms of both middle fingers touch as the other fingers intertwine.

Figure 9.1. Inju: The art of longevity (part two)

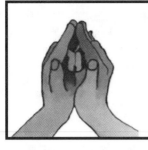

Fatigue-Releasing lnju #2
The midlle fingernails meet as the middle fingers bend toward each other. The palms of the remaining fingers are erect and touching.

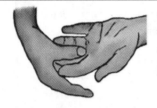

Fatigue-Releasing lnju #3
The pad of the thumb touches the base of the middle finger on the opposite hand, palm side.

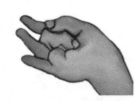

Fatigue-Releasing lnju #4
The midlle finger bends into the pad of the thumb on the same hand
while the thumb rests on the top of the bent middle finger.

Figure 9.1. Inju: The art of longevity (part three)

The Sacred Sites of the body reveal the story of embryogenesis, or human prenatal evolution. They tell us how we have come to be who we are in literal, practical, physiological, and energetic terms. They are the keys to the master plan of formative development. When we recharge these sacred sites through touch and awareness, we awaken our chosen birthright of embodiment. Embodiment occurs not only in the physical form but also at the soul level. To be embodied is to be vital, healthy, strong, and focused with undying trust and confidence in the manifestation of soul purpose. This is the promise of the Master Plan. It is completely reliable.

THE EMBRYOGENESIS OF THE SACRED SITES:
EMBRYOLOGICAL PROCESSES

SACRED SITE	ASCENDING OR DESCENDING	FUNCTION	EMBRYOLOGICAL PROCESS	PRENATAL TIME— IN UTERO
#1	Descending	The Prime Mover, Awakening, the Initiator, Movement	Fertilization and conception; development from one cell to sixteen cells	Days 1–7 first week
High 1		The Mover's Support, Confidence, Encouragement, Trust in Action		
#2	Ascending	Wisdom, Intuition, Vision, Inspiration	Implantation; development of neural groove	Days 8–13 second week
#3	Ascending	Respiration, Receptivity, Breath	Vasculature; beginnings of differentiation of heart and brain from the same tissue	Days 14–20 third week
#4*	Ascending	Shamanic Gateway, Consciousness	Optic structures; rapid cranial development; differentiation of cranial nerves, spinal cord, and brain stem; by the end of fourth week of gestation the entire blueprint and foundation for the vertebral column and its discs, supporting soft tissue, vascular system, and nerve supply are in place	Days 21–27 fourth week

*SPECIAL NOTE: Sacred Site #4 is a major growth juncture. Energetically this is when the "spark of life" ignites due to the establishment of consciousness through neurobiological networking. From this point on the baby is said to have a midline—a central channel both physiologically and energetically.

THE EMBRYOGENESIS OF THE SACRED SITES:
EMBRYOLOGICAL PROCESSES (CONT.)

SACRED SITE	ASCENDING OR DESCENDING	FUNCTION	EMBRYOLOGICAL PROCESS	PRENATAL TIME— IN UTERO
#5	Descending	Adrenal Support, Fearless	Kidneys develop along with intestinal loop	Days 28–33
#6	Descending	Balance, "the Chiropractic," Structural Integrity	Trunk elongates and strengthens	Days 34–37
#7	Ascending	Peace or Peace Bridge, the Crossroads, Victory, Death and Rebirth	Eyelids and toes develop	Days 38–44
#8	Ascending	Alchemy, Clarity	Intestines almost complete; dental areas prepared; hands and feet can contact each other	Days 45–56 completion of the second month
Low 8		The Purgative, the Dispeller, the Alchemist's Assistant		

Content created by Stephanie Mines, Ph.D.,
The TARA Approach for the Resolution of Shock and Trauma, 2006.

THE EMBRYOGENESIS OF THE SACRED SITES:
FETAL PROCESSES

From week 9/Sacred Site #9 onward the baby is known as a fetus.
Organogenesis is fundamentally complete.

SACRED SITE	ASCENDING OR DESCENDING	FUNCTION	FETAL PROCESS	PRENATAL TIME— IN UTERO
#9	Ascending	Transition, Space, the End of One Cycle and the Beginning of Another	Placenta forms; sexual organs differentiate; face has human profile; liver develops; waste products are eliminated	Weeks 9–12
#10		Transformation, Voice, Expression, the Beginning of a New Cycle		
#11		Unloading, the Yoke, Independence		
#12		Surrender, Body Truth		
#13	Descending	The Mother, Integration, Calm, Serenity	Coordinated movements occur; body fattens and grows rapidly; absorbing nourishment and developing fleshy protection; further differentiation of genitalia	Weeks 13–15
#14		The Sustainer, the Assimilator		
#15		Wash Your Heart with Laughter, Joy in Everything		
#16	Ascending	The Foundation, Muscular Joy, Resilience, Youthfulness	Activity; movement; eyes and ears find their definitive position; ovaries reach full development	Week 16

THE EMBRYOGENESIS OF THE SACRED SITES:
FETAL PROCESSES (CONT.)

SACRED SITE	ASCENDING OR DESCENDING	FUNCTION	FETAL PROCESS	PRENATAL TIME— IN UTERO
#17	Ascending	The Connector, Unity, Nervous System, Harmony	Growth slows down during this period as the fetal body stabilizes; protective vernix is produced and covers the body for protection	Week 17
#18	Descending	The Pathmaker	Feet reach final development; increased protection for the fetus is provided by lanugo;* eyebrows and head hair develop; fetal body develops a fatty adipose tissue that produces protective heat; the bones of the skull and the middle ear appear; nervous system is developing rapidly, particularly in the 20th week; myelin formation in the spinal cord and nerve roots begins; messages from the brain are clearly transmitted through nerve fiber tracts (the corticospinal fiber tracts)	Weeks 18–20
#19		Being in the Center of Your Own Life, Boundaries		
High 19		Selfhood, Really Good Boundries		
#20		Conscious Awakening, Genius		
#21	Descending	True Security, Freedom from Worry, Reliever of Mental Chaos	Substantial weight gain occurs; body proportions, including facial arrangement, are established in their final forms	Weeks 21–22
#22		Contentment, Adaptation, Wholeness in the Moment, Be Here Now		

*Lanugo is a fine downy hair that covers the body, strengthening the function of the vernix.

SACRED SITE	ASCENDING OR DESCENDING	FUNCTION	FETAL PROCESS	PRENATAL TIME— IN UTERO
#23	Ascending	Destiny, Patience, Rest in the Order of the Order	Maturation of the central nervous system; increasing weight gain and brain development; lungs capable of postnatal respiration; an upright stance becomes structurally possible (6th month onward); all the neurons within the central nervous system are present by the beginning of the 7th month; neural circuits specialize; all brain cells are present before delivery	Weeks 23–38
#24		Peacemaker, Relationship Counselor		
#25		Regeneration		
#26		Self-Love, Completion		

Content created by Stephanie Mines, Ph.D.,
The TARA Approach for the Resolution of Shock and Trauma, 2006.

REWILDING OURSELVES:
SENSORY ACUITY AND RESILIENCE

We do not have to be exact. We just need to listen to our bodies. Our bodies are exact.

MARY IINO BURMEISTER

Trauma and shock force us inward into a focus on sensory tracking that appears, amid being overwhelmed, to be a separation from the present and a fracturing of self. Simultaneous with those consequences, however, is an immersion in the somatic world of sensory acuity. This resembles, and often fully replicates, the world of the embryo.

The sensory acuity of embryonic life that is so highly responsive to and interactive with all environmental dimensions is a state of thorough somatic engagement. Once we acquire language and are held to the rules of behavior in our culture and family, that degree of sensory presence and orientation is no longer well received. Most of us shape up fairly readily and exchange the sensory-dominant compass for a more rational, logical, and behaviorally acceptable style of orientation.

True healing draws us back into the sensory world to learn the language of our feelings. The more we can be present to our sensory reports, the more we reclaim Original Brilliance. Original Brilliance is Embryonic Intelligence. The pulse-listening that is central to the Art of Compassion is an utterly somatic approach to listening deeply to Embryonic Intelligence. When we palpate the Sacred Sites with our fingertips we hear the story, in pulsation or embryonic language, of each site. This is sensory tracking of the highest order. It tells the energetic story of how we survived, and it shows us our way home. It is the energetic physiology of the Wounded Healer.

Most of the people whom I ask to tell me about their prenatal life or their birth—and I ask almost everyone about this—say they don't remember. The majority respond with incredulity to my query as if I should have known their answer already since the assumption is that no one can remember that early time. Yet what I know is actually the opposite. I know without doubt that the full story of embryogenesis is available to each one of us.

Each of the Sacred Sites tells their segment in the sequence of the epic saga of unique human development. The site stories are particular to each individual. Of course you remember. You made it all happen. Restoring the bounty of sensory wisdom that is archived in connective tissue is the pathway to regeneration and one of the secrets of resilience. The following stories illustrate that, beginning with one that remains especially stunning to me.

Even with my enormous faith in the human capacity to remember the details of early life, I would have been skeptical about Diana's experience if I had not witnessed it myself.

DIANA AND THE MYSTERY OF MEMORY

Psychic energy is indomitable. Even when crushed, it rises like a phoenix. It transcends the density of the body, even though physical form is its vehicle.

STEPHANIE MINES

Diana was adopted very soon after her birth, within hours. It was an adoption arranged even while she was in utero. She grew up in a middle-class family on the East Coast of the United States. Her adoptive parents only revealed they had adopted her when Diana was on the verge of young adulthood, preparing to enter a prestigious master's in business administration program to which she had been granted a full scholarship.

She took the information about being adopted in stride. She never felt particularly close to either of her parents or her brother. It turns out they were both adopted. They learned about their adoption together in a family meeting in which everyone agreed it would take some time to absorb the news. The absence of emotional affect was their comfort zone.

Diana met me much later when, as a flourishing entrepreneur, she struggled with severe allergies and was referred to me by her physician. Her physical ailments did not impede her success in any way because she would not allow them to do that, but they did make her wonder about her birth parents and her genetic inheritance. After all, she might want to have children one day. Due to various legal barricades, she had not, at the time we met, been able to contact her biological parents.

Immunity is a facet of identity. It is the composite signature of genetic, epigenetic, and exposome lettering. These are added to the particular compensations, sensorily registered and calibrated to reflect strategies to overcome survival threats, that each person generates. Every individual's immune response is a database, a nervous system track record.

Diana and I undertook together a creative, ingenious approach to bypassing the legal roadblocks to her birth records by asking her cellular matrix and her connective tissue for the answers that bureaucracies refused to provide. What happened stunned us with its accuracy. Everything her body told us was later corroborated when the roadblocks were taken down and Diana was able to contact her birth mother.

In addition to troublesome allergies and food sensitivities, Diana was irritated by another unresolved dilemma in her life. She had not found a life partner. Financially solvent, resourceful, inventive, athletic, and attractive, she was single and not happy about it. Diana had a real love of relationship, and she was generously available for it. This case study originates in the pre-pandemic era, so it includes events in which people met in person. All of my first interactions with Diana were in person, though I remain a resource for her post-pandemic, online. Being the innovative thinker she is, Diana wondered if she could connect the allergies with a way in which she may have acquired an allergy to intimacy.

Diana and I collaborated to explore her questions in a series of meetings over a week that was entirely devoted to her healing. In the Art of Compassion there is a template called the Five-Day Intensive. This is a process whereby deep investigations into the origins of distress can be explored. I look to causation at the source level, from the first moment of exposure to all the opportunists that threaten Original Brilliance and Embryonic Intelligence. Diana agreed to pursue that approach, which was why she had chosen me to accompany her in her research.

Accompany is the correct word because in the Five-Day Intensive journey, or in any context like it, I follow much more than lead. There is always awe and amazement in the process of following. Surprises abound.

In this case, though, the awe was at a higher order of magnitude because of the detail in which Diana was able to remember the circumstances and the people who were her vehicle of becoming. The specifics were so exact that she continually questioned them, but in the end, they were undeniable, and finally proved beyond doubt. At this time Diana had none of the stories about her parents' meeting and relationship and her mother's pregnancy with her that some people are told. It was all a tabula rasa. This made what unfolded during our week together stunning.

During our Five-Day Intensive immersion, Diana and I explored how energy medicine, particularly as self-care, could be a resource for her to diminish, if not completely eliminate, the discomfort, itchiness, fatigue, and fuzzy-headedness of her allergic responses. We looked at her skin eruptions with the same goal—to experiment with hands-on self-care applications that she could apply at the onset of allergic reactions. Diana was new to the concepts of energy medicine and the ongoing self-care discipline. She was experiencing some breathing restriction, which usually preceded an allergic response, and a prickly rash had begun. This was good experimental material. We tried a variety of options.

One application was particularly soothing. It involved simply holding the right and left sides of the base of the sternum where Sacred Site #14 is located.

This site manages assimilation. It also is embodying. Furthermore, it assists in integrating destabilizing feelings like enormous rage or grief. Diana found that when she held this area she could breathe more easily, but she also felt very sad. I commented on her sensory acuity, which I believe is a hallmark of the Wounded Healer.

We also used the Rediscovery Journey template. Diana had very clear images of her birth mother during the Rediscovery process. Diana had the sense that her mother was in a toxic environment in which she felt trapped, almost imprisoned. It was shattering. Diana questioned herself. Where could these images be coming from? I encouraged her to trust them with an experimental perspective. I joined her in mutual curiosity.

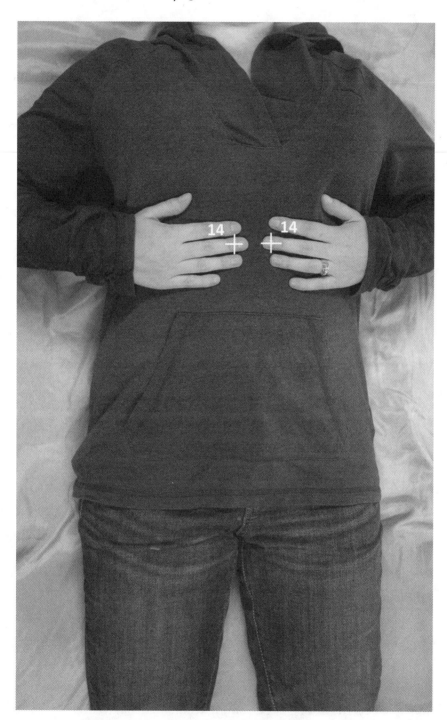

Figure 9.2. Sacred Site #14

It is one thing to read research about how and where memory is stored and quite another to witness and be party to the experience of knowing, beyond a doubt, that memory is available throughout the body. When does memory about particular experiences surface, and why does it manifest when it does? This has been explored in so many ways, from scientific studies, including by the Nobel prize–winning Dr. Eric Kandel, to the novels of Marcel Proust, who coined the phrase "involuntary memory." To experience memory emerging as coherent, visual, and completely accurate depictions when the one remembering has no logical access to that information, is like witnessing a psychic event even though it is science at work.

We continued to excavate remarkable memories during the Five-Day Intensive, which combined hands-on energy medicine and the Rediscovery Journey. Several years later, when Diana was pregnant with her first child, she was given access to her birth records. She went with her husband to meet her birth mother in Michigan. It wasn't on their first meeting, but after a while, when they felt they had some degree of ease with each other, Diana's mother told her about being confined during her pregnancy in a place that was later condemned for asbestos and lead paint. She said she had thought about that over and over. Had the paint affected the baby she gave up for adoption?

By reclaiming our earliest history, we have access to increased self-respect and admiration for the stalwart, unflagging devotion to life that sustains us. We dared all then, and we risked all for life.

Diana and her birth mother explored the possibility of detoxification, even so many years later, from the environmental contaminants that they absorbed. They used a combination of energy medicine from the TARA Approach, as well as herbal and dietary resources, and they were successful in significantly reducing inflammatory responses in their bodies. By doing this together they forged a bond between them that was unique and lasting. Everyone benefits when intergenerational healing happens. Each iteration is a song for the family of the Earth.

NATASHA AND THE DIRECTORY
OF PRENATAL HURDLES

Your silence is almost worst of all.

GRETA THUNBERG,
NO ONE IS TOO SMALL TO MAKE A DIFFERENCE

Natasha was conceived under the most horrific of circumstances: a violent rape. Yet despite an atmosphere of unwantedness, she survived. Her life outside the womb was even more difficult. She showed signs of not thriving. But she made it. Her near-extinction experiences shaped her commitment to being a voice for our living Earth and for all species threatened with extinction.

Natasha's story exemplifies how healing from trauma and going beyond trauma to wholeness is a natural process. Healing from trauma has become an industry, like almost everything in the West. Nevertheless, the most effective trauma therapist has always been Mother Nature, the natural world. When I was researching secondary traumatization and interviewing veterans and their families, one gentleman shared with me his experience. It resonates with Natasha's story. This man, let's call him Ernie, spoke to me about how the therapists he had seen and the pharmaceuticals they recommended, along with everything else they offered, seemed to result in an ongoing worsening of his condition. He became so unbearable that his wife and children were threatening to either boot him out of the house or leave themselves. That is when Ernie made a turning-point decision.

Before his military service Ernie had purchased a piece of wilderness land on which he had always hoped to construct a vacation home for his family. Now he decided to go onto that land and build a small cabin, by hand, and by himself. This choice was his breakthrough to wholeness. It took almost a year, but by the time Ernie was done with building his cabin, he was rooted, vitalized, mended, sane, healthy, sober, and grateful. He returned to his wife and children for truth and reconciliation. He was regenerated by the Master Healer. I will never forget Ernie's story, nor will I ever forget Natasha's.

My vocation as a trauma therapist has opened a window into the most exhilarating and the most brutal aspects of the human experience. Brutality to innocent children is excruciating to hear about, much less experience. As an unwanted child Natasha had been battered in every conceivable way. As she grew up, surviving daily oppression and viciousness, she found refuge in plants, trees, and animals. Her blessing was that she had access to the natural world, and she capitalized on that at every opportunity.

The beauty was that she never questioned her deep communication with the nonhuman world. This was her source of sanity and self-regulation. The fortitude, sensory acuity, clarity, and perseverance of this young being are a wonder. It is also innate, organic, and completely understandable. We are all extraordinary.

It was because Natasha knew firsthand what it meant to face extinction that she became such a determined, focused, and authentic climate activist and animal rights advocate. It is in this context that I met her. She was a student of Regenerative Health as a methodology for self-care along with other climate activists and was one of my first students to adapt the TARA Approach for animals and encouraged me to include them. She was one of the first of my students to study with me completely online. She represents a new era of technology-savvy youth who have a heightened sensitivity to the natural world, a deep sense of urgency about the climate crisis, and the capacity to wield technology as an instrument for the evolution of consciousness.

I am in awe of how trauma survivors become unprecedented leaders. No matter how much I know and share about the path of the Wounded Healer, I remain humbled by the generosity of spirit that pours forth from those who have endured the greatest evil. Natasha is one of those who may call me her teacher, but I am her student. She told me about her breakthrough, her leap beyond trauma. She described it as an eruption—a sudden and spontaneous blooming. It was, she said, the volcanic explosion of her destiny. It came, fully formed, out of being crushed and ground down until something had to give; something had to be alchemized from the rubble of what was done to her. She arose from that rubble like a deity burnished by abrasive forces and then polished so that the true metal of her selfhood was evident.

Natasha had another mentor, in addition to Mother Earth. This was, and is, Greta Thunberg, the young Swedish climate activist who has taken the world by storm by speaking truth to power. It was Greta Thunberg who helped instill in Natasha the confidence that her goal of rousing a groundswell of activists to turn the climate crisis around was feasible. It was Greta's daring disclosure of her loneliness and withdrawal that spurred Natasha to explore how she could transmute her own tendency to isolate.

She suddenly knew that she could counter the mounting evidence pointing to the fact that extinction was inevitable. Natasha had been there herself. Her extinction was inevitable, and she turned it around.

Greta Thunberg did not have a history of attempted annihilation by her own parents, like Natasha had, but nevertheless, Natasha felt that Greta had the lived experience of hopelessness and despair that came with that early shock and trauma.

As Natasha walked among the ancient pines of the Caledonian rain forest, near to her home in Scotland, she would stop and pick up the needles she found on the ropey, leaf-covered earth. Rubbing these between her fingers she would breathe in what she felt was certainly a rare medicine because of how it uplifted her spirits. She was certain it was this medicine that empowered her to salvage her will from the alcoholic rages and attacks that were part of her daily life at home. The threatened rape of this land she loved, a land that conveyed the history of the Earth and the history of the bond between humans and the natural world, was unthinkable—intolerable. She would not allow it.

Passion rose in her like a Primordial Fire. It kept her alive. It gave her direction. She would use every ounce of vitality she could muster to prevent the death sentence of ignorance and unconsciousness.

At the first moment that Natasha was able to separate from her parents and live independently, she did. She arranged her life so that she could prioritize her activism. She became friends with like-minded people and joined organizations like Extinction Rebellion and Rights of Nature. She campaigned against ecocide. She sat in circles in which people talked about sustainability and regeneration and how they could find the internal reserve to persevere in what was surely a lengthy effort. She engaged in conversations about inner climate, personal trauma, and how these played a role in climate activism. She participated in direct action.

Natasha told me that it was reading the index of likely thresholds of pre- and perinatal shock that awakened her to the magnitude of her courage and intelligence. She realized that she had invested everything she had in order to be alive in this movement. This was the beginning of her self-respect and self-honoring.

I include that index here, albeit in an abbreviated form, at Natasha's encouragement, and the encouragement of my own embryonic self, so that my readers can have the opportunity to experience what Natasha describes. One caveat, however: titrate the pace of reading. If you feel stirred to reflect and journal, or do whatever will promote integration, please do so. Take your time.

❧

ABBREVIATED DIRECTORY OF PRENATAL AND PERINATAL PSYCHOLOGY LANDMARKS

Anesthesia

When anesthesia is administered to a woman in labor the dosage is based on her weight. Thus, the baby is always overdosed.

In their book *Ghosts from the Nursery,* Robin Karr-Morse and Meredith Wiley report that "studies indicate that the use of obstetrical anesthesia during delivery may cause subtle alterations in the formation of neurons, synapses, and neural transmitters that are undetectable at birth. One seven-year study of over three thousand babies showed long-lasting effects of anesthesia on behavior and motor development."

Birth Stages

Stage One: Initiation

Stage one is the initiatory cycle in the birthing process. It is when the baby has intimations of change and makes the first hormonal gestures toward launching the journey through the birth canal. This can be a tenuous, determined, fearful, or confusing time. Needless to say, all previous in utero experiences lay the groundwork for initiation.

The physical simulations of initiation are also new experiences. Hormones are aroused that are purposeful, designed to fuel the necessities of birth.

Stage Two: Navigation

Once the initiatory phase occurs, the next challenge for the baby is navigation. The shape of the mother's pelvis is a crucial determining factor, as is how the baby's movements forward implicate the umbilical cord. A narrow pelvis can exert restrictive pressures, making the baby feel suffocated. The umbilical cord can entwine the baby's body in any number of ways to impede or even completely halt movement. The protruding lumbosacral promontory can pose a significant navigational obstacle, requiring flexibility and creativity.

Neurological development in utero is organized to promote skill at navigation. It is also organized to promote muscular and energetic attunement between mother and child.

Stage two may happen for mother and baby in the hospital. The

fear the mother may feel there, or anywhere, can send confusing mes-
sages to the navigating baby. Adrenaline antidotes oxytocin. Oxytocin
is the hormone that drives the progression of labor, so when oxytocin is
antidoted, labor halts.

When labor halts, medical professionals tend to introduce chemical
stimulants rather than directing attention to relaxing Mom. Pitocin or
other stimulants are used to jump-start labor, sometimes detrimentally,
as moms can have abreactions. When labor is no longer being directed
by a baby, navigation becomes difficult. It is like trying to steer your car
when you are drunk or drugged.

Stage Three: Presentation

This stage, which refers to the first appearance of the baby outside the
womb, is about being seen. Responses to presentations have an immediate effect on the child's confidence and self-esteem. Direct, welcoming
contact with the mother and father, whenever possible, and skin-to-skin
connection is optimum. If siblings can be present, all the better.
Immediate eye contact with Mom is the highest priority.

Generally, this leads to what can be described as "people shock" or
"need shock." We cannot trust, and we are unclear about how to get our
needs met when these conditions prevail.

Breach, Cesarean, and Twin Presentations

All the conditions discussed in this directory of primary obstacles
encountered from conception through birth apply to those born in the
breach position, delivered by cesarean, and also to twins.

In addition, breach presentations may be a demonstration of Divine
Homesickness as the baby is oriented, as if going back instead of ahead.
It is important to support the breach baby's unique approaches.

Cesarean deliveries are disempowering for both mother and child.
This can be repatterned by creating the opportunity to sequence the
powerful drives associated with birth. There are many games that

babies and children can play to help them complete their birth experiences. These games can also be played by anyone at any age!

- Make birth tunnels and let babies scramble through them, to be met on the other side with applause, celebration, and hugs.
- Make your way through turtleneck sweaters, zippered-up vests, and similar garments, celebrating the head's emergence.
- Swing, emphasizing the victory of coming forward to a waiting face(s) with the intention of empowering the capacity to move forward.

In twin births, each child's experience can be treated individually, while at the same time comprehending the shared dynamics of their cohabitation and the effect of the decisions made in utero for successful emergence.

Conception

Conception is the first lesson in the realm of form and matter. Imagine arriving somewhere after a long journey. Perhaps you have traveled for hours, or even days, by plane or car or bus. How are you met when you arrive? Are you given a soft place to rest? Are you provided with sustenance and refreshment? Or are you not even recognized by those you have come to see? Are you left alone, without comfort or companionship? These are the variables of conception shock. They affect our sense of safety, worth, and value. Personality and behavior are built upon how we compensate for and survive this test of physical, embodied manifestation.

Discovery

The term *discovery* refers to the recognition by the mother that a child is present within her. The precise time when discovery occurs varies.

Some women realize they are with child at the moment they

conceive. Others sense the presence of their baby even before conception. In many ways the earliest discovery is optimum, as it provides support for manifestation. It validates the journey from non-differentiation to substance, just as birth marks the transition from prenatal life to postnatal life. Being welcomed at these transitions encourages health.

From the biochemical standpoint, cells begin to pump signals to the mother in the first days after fertilization. When the embryo is embedded in the womb (implantation), these chemical messengers multiply.

The secretion of the hormone called HCG (human chorionic gonadotropin) speaks clearly of the presence of a successfully embedded embryo. HCG initiates a hormonal cascade in the mother's body, prodding it to secrete progesterone so that menstruation will not begin. This is the most common signal of discovery.

Divine Homesickness

Divine Homesickness is the dominating feeling that one does not belong here on this Earth at this time. People who have this feeling sense there is somewhere else they should be. This place is usually purer, more undifferentiated, nondualistic, and sensitive.

In relationships, people with Divine Homesickness prolong the romantic honeymoon aspect with an emphasis on merging rather than differentiating and maturing. They may prefer animals and nature to contact with people, because both animals and nature are more unconditional than humans.

Divine Homesickness is infused with grief at the loss of a more heavenly realm, or it may be rage that dominates the feeling of exile to the Earth plane. Feeling trapped in the body is the signature of Divine Homesickness.

Egg and Sperm Memory

We all have cellular memories of the energetic, emotional, and psychological energies present at our conception. Those maintaining the paradigm that memory must be cognitive will likely find this statement ludicrous. However, it is nevertheless true that we have an innate knowledge of the male and female contributions to our being. These memories may be subtle and fleeting, imagistic, metaphoric, and dreamlike until we focus on them and claim them as our history. Egg and sperm, like all life, have intelligence, and the nature of intelligence is to communicate itself.

Every emotion and biochemical change associated with emotion in parents affects development from conception onward. These attributes are implicit in the egg and sperm contributions to conception. Changes in stress hormones, such as cortisol and epinephrine, create neurochemical cascades that shape immune function and all health. Neurotransmitters circulated in the parents' bodies imprint neurological information. This is how learning is retained implicitly. Minute changes in hormones affect cell growth. Beginning with conception, the child is growing its nervous system, brain, and organs—while swimming in a biochemical soup.

Forceps and Suction

While forceps are not used with the same frequency today as in the past, they are still in use. In some places they have been replaced by suction or other means of forcible extraction.

The effect of a forceps or suction delivery on the baby is mitigated by the intention with which they are used. With loving intention and communication, the experience can be changed from invasion to support.

Cranial treatment right after delivery can erase the damages of manipulation of the baby's head at birth. Birth is a highly compressive experience. The compressive forces help shape the developing cranium, but they can also be damaging. There are times when the use of forceps or suction can be lifesaving. At these times the arriving baby can be informed of what is about to happen, and all applications can be infused with loving-kindness.

Without intention and loving-kindness, the use of forceps translates as a power struggle that the baby must lose. Rage is a common response to this losing battle.

Implantation and the Great Placenta

Implantation describes the process by which the embryo completely embeds itself in the endometrium. It occurs during the first week after conception.

Implantation is thoroughly completed by the second week in utero. Within twelve days the embryo has burrowed into the uterine endometrium. This is a major embryonic task.

Implantation leads, virtually simultaneously, to the creation of the placenta. The fetus contributes significantly by making antigens on the placental surface that completely block any rejection by the mother. In more than fifty years of research, no one has been able to explain why the mother's body does not reject the placenta. What occurs at this crucial stage of life defies all the laws of immunology and transplantation.

Loss

Loss makes its mark on tissue. Scarring is a hieroglyphic, and the cave drawings on the womb are read by the inhabitants. When a child is lost, either through abortion, miscarriage, the result of an accident, a chromosomal abnormality, twin loss, or any reason whatsoever, the story of that loss indwells the mother's body and meets the conceptus.

Social Engagement

The social engagement system consists of the cranial nerves that insert at the base of the skull. These nerves direct our spontaneous interaction with others through the eyes, by listening to what others say and responding appropriately, through reaching out and making healthy physical contact, and by enjoying community and relationship. If the people responsible for us when we are small fail to protect us; are aggressive, violating, or violent toward us; or if they disappoint, reject, or abandon us, the social engagement system and the cranial nerves suffer. Generally, this leads to what can be described as "people shock" or "need shock." We cannot trust, and we are unclear about how to get our needs met when these conditions prevail.

Toxicity

Pregnancy is a porous time, and the world communicates with the developing baby through the mother's body. Environmental toxins can penetrate in a variety of ways. Cigarette smoke, for instance, can create a pervasively toxic environment for a developing being. Toxins can also be emotions, ideas, stressors, and expectations. Toxins come through the umbilical cord, like cigarette smoke, alcohol, drugs, contaminants in foods and fluids, and environmental toxins, as well as through what the baby hears and sees.

Trimester Hallmarks

Each trimester is marked by certain hallmarks. The hallmarks of the first environment chart presented earlier in the book (see figure 9.3) as well as the embryogenesis chart (see the tables on pages 117–21) provide some of this detail.

The first trimester is the most spacious experience.

The second trimester is a time of intensive learning as sensory perceptions of sound, sight, and touch are amplified.

The third trimester is the most intensive period of preparation for the marathon of navigation and presentation. All the trimesters are training periods, but I think of the third trimester as training for a triathlon. Babies fatten up for the big output of labor and grow their brains to become the most precise navigation system possible.

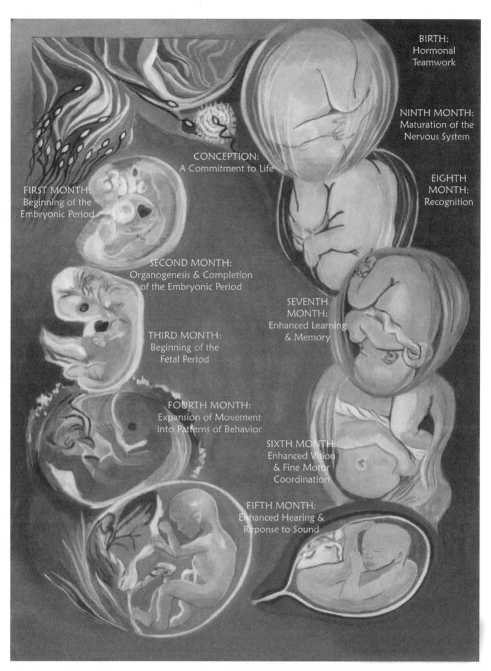

Figure 9.3. Hallmarks of the
first environment

Twin Loss

Twin loss refers to the experience in utero of losing a twin, at any stage of pregnancy or at birth. This is known to happen with greater frequency than was previously reported. Twin loss can go undetected by parents, particularly when it occurs early in pregnancy.

Unwantedness

Unwantedness is surely one of the most severe forms of shock. Deplorable conditions of various kinds are usually the backdrop to unwantedness. There are varying degrees of unwantedness, and these can shift during pregnancy. The most extreme form of unwantedness is annihilation ideation, or the intention that the child not survive. There can also be fleeting moments of unwantedness in any pregnancy. This spectrum must be considered in evaluating the experience of unwantedness.

EMBRYONIC INTELLIGENCE
AND UNPRECEDENTED LEADERSHIP

Embryonic Intelligence is the realization that you are always at the beginning.

STEPHANIE MINES

Conception shock, discovery shock, the pain of unwantedness: Natasha knew it all, and she knew it somatically. She was not stunned by the descriptions she read. On the contrary, they relieved her. She felt seen in the words that described what she knew in her body to be her experience. She could drop her guardedness now. There was not something wrong with her. In fact, she was an amazing, incredible, courageous being. She could be present to others, as Greta Thunberg was now.

Natasha realized in every cell of her being that she was a child of the Earth. Those Caledonian pines were redolent with the scent of her true mother line. Like them, she felt an indomitable commitment to being upright, protective, and enduring. She had survived and come into her own wholeness to be a voice for our living Earth. What could possibly be more important than that?

Embryonic Intelligence is sensory, exploratory, fully present, and unconditional. It is one of the secrets of resilience. Though squashed, suppressed, minimized, disregarded, patronized, and misunderstood, it never dies. When we reclaim it and attribute to it the respect and value that is its due, we move beyond trauma. We breakthrough to inhabit the wholeness that is our organizational principle. This always happens in concert with the natural world. Even if you live, as I did, in a tenement in the Bronx, the natural world finds its way to you and you to it, through whatever means possible.

Truly unprecedented leadership arises from Embryonic Intelligence and ignites the evolution of consciousness. Because Embryonic Intelligence is always in the mode of differentiation, it leans in to the unknown, the ever-present mystery, with courage and as part of a unified field of consciousness—never singular, always collaborative.

10
The Secret of Resilience

Embryonic Intelligence is Interbeing. It is the unified field of consciousness.

STEPHANIE MINES

Embryonic Intelligence, the spark of Original Brilliance that is constantly beginning, constantly differentiating, is available to anyone at any time throughout life. It is not a course or a webinar. It is your birthright and always has been. By *embryonic* I do not mean only the intelligence of the embryo at the time of embryogenesis. I refer to the state of consciousness that is embryonic originality. This is somatic consciousness. It is the newness and purity of sensory presence in intimate, interactive kinship with the total environment—including the unseen. This is the overarching secret to resilience. The characteristics of this secret are further elucidated in this chapter.

Adult development built on compensations for the thwarted full expression of original, embryonic, and differentiated brilliance is our downfall. It is responsible for the climate crisis and its associated crises, including the COVID-19 pandemic. Compensatory, separated, and hierarchical, us-and-them strategizing is colonial, extractive, and usury, even if it appears to be successful. Embryonic Intelligence is consistently unifying, collective, and inclusive. It is without ego. Ego itself is compensation for the horrific, fragmenting, and disorienting pain of disconnection. That disconnection is everyone's first and most debilitating, overwhelming shock. The time has come to move beyond it.

Embryonic Intelligence is highly varied, bursting with vibrant, even scintillating personality, on a broad spectrum of diverse—including neurodiverse—manifestations. The daring to step forward, to be seen as a unique, whole being, sheltered in the protective arms of personal destiny, like the aura of the corona radiata (the inner glycoprotein layer that guards the ovum). This protective field is ours when we reclaim the energy of embryonic, Original Brilliance. Once liberated, Embryonic Intelligence will continually unfold, just as the embryo unfolds. It guides us and we follow it, using our honed sensory acuity.

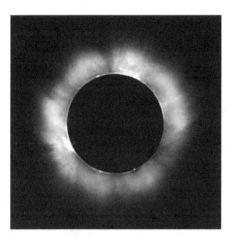

Figure 10.1. Corona radiata

CORONA RADIATA

Embryonic Intelligence weaves sensory acuity and differentiation into every life moment. This is not a product you get somewhere. You cannot order it online. It does not cost anything. We already have it; it was always there. It does, however, get buried. I am eternally grateful to the transmission of the simple, profound wisdoms, such as what I learned about the Art of Compassion, that continually remove layers from the falsities piled needlessly onto Embryonic Intelligence and expose Original Brilliance. It is largely that gratitude that inspires this book, in partnership with the unfolding of my own embryonic guidance.

I uncovered the secret to resilience—Embryonic Intelligence and Original Brilliance—independent of anyone's instruction or direction. It is my own evolutionary way forward, revealed to me by my inner compass. I now know it is the force of being that keeps me here despite my frequent doubts about the value of my existence. It fuels my commitment to being and, by extension, to everyone else's. It contains the crystalline clarity about my own frequently remarkable (to me) endurance. It sparks my determination to be of service, just as trees are of service in their stalwart holding of space, their communications with each other, and their unconditional, enduring, and witnessing memory systems. I want to honor Suzanne Simard here for her courageous research and devotion to her own Original Brilliance, which kept her going so she could share the model of the Mother Trees for us to emulate. Her book, *Finding the Mother Tree,* wherein she weaves her personal story with her seminal, watershed research inspired me to do a similar weaving in this book.

An alchemical awakening occurs when we see through the eyes of our embryonic selves. This is the vision that is prophetic. It imparts certainty in being, even if, as is so often the case, Original Brilliance is rejected, cornered, obfuscated, or disregarded. Once Original Brilliance is exposed, given space, and nurtured, its buoyancy is dependable. Indeed, buoyancy is the nature of embryonic, Original Brilliance. It cannot be deflated. It will always bounce back. Discovering this for yourself is the true resolution of trauma, and, as the stories of Ernie and Natasha illustrate, it can occur through communion with nature as the Master Therapist.

There is something organically psychedelic about this awakening to Original Brilliance. As Sally Gillespie says in *Climate Crisis and Consciousness,* "Seeing ourselves as a part of our ecosystems, local and global, induces an Alice in Wonderland experience of feeling both smaller and bigger than our habitual selves." We have, in the laboratories of our bodies, our own pharmacy of psychedelics. They are stored in the cabinet marked "consciousness," and climate change opens that cabinet for us if we allow it. I can say with confidence that the natural world encourages us to open that cabinet. Embryonic Intelligence is ubiquitous and linked with the eternal. It is our clue to meeting the climate crisis, and it also transcends the climate crisis.

Components of the Secret of Resilience

Embryonic, Original Brilliance

Sensory Acuity
Differentiation
Voicing Truth: Articulating Original Brilliance
Kinship with the Natural World
Ongoing Emergence

SENSORY ACUITY

Creation is not just at the beginning; it is the ongoing ever-present energy assuming temporary patterns in the physical body within each present moment.

MARY IINO BURMEISTER

Sensory acuity is the hallmark of Embryonic Intelligence. It is what is meant by pure, complete presence. This is the brilliance in little ones we are magnetized to but find unwieldy, sometimes even diagnosable, in grown-ups. Sensory acuity speaks in the language of the natural world. When we follow sensory awareness, it takes us much further in the direction of innovation than is even possible for cognitive processes. Sensory acuity is intimately aligned with intuition, creativity, and imagination. This is what Albert Einstein was referring to when he said, "The intuitive mind is a sacred gift, and the rational mind is a faithful servant. We have created a society that honors the servant and has forgotten the gift." This is the time to correct that error. Embryonic Intelligence is the intuitive mind. It is not reserved for geniuses like Einstein. He is a model of surrendering to the sacred gift and celebrating it. This is a model anyone who is willing to surrender can follow.

Sensory acuity means noticing and then tracking sensory experiences. The tracking is what we can do as adults that we did not need to do as little ones. Eventually the tracking clarifies patterns of sensation that can then be translated into intuitive guidance. There is always a quality of mystery about this guidance. Once again, I reference Albert Einstein, who said, "At times I feel certain that I am right while not knowing the reason." Once you can feel (meaning sense) what certainty is, then confidence is readily available with or without the rational data, which may, or may not, come later.

The practice of sensory acuity, or sensory tracking, and the capacity to see the patterns in your own unique sensory orchestration will enforce the dominance and eventual triumph of Original Brilliance. We need to practice this because of how much we have been entrained in the error that Einstein references in his statement about the gift and the servant.

The story I tell in the beginning of this book about following the demanding sensory experiences that led me to a breakthrough discovery about my prenatal life is an example of sensory tracking. Indeed, we do that tracking when we are in pain or at risk. At those moments we are bonded with sensation. That is the model that we can adapt when we are not threatened and use it to access the stunning innovations that occur when our sensory systems link with executive function, surpassing what was possible when we were brilliant, sensory-oriented toddlers.

We read stories about rising above threats all the time, like the passenger on a train who reaches her hand out to a killer who shows up with a knife, or the woman who offers a sandwich to a thief who has broken into her home. These miraculous tales are the result of sensory tracking—following the sensory guidance that is Original Brilliance and that saves lives by illuminating a truth deeper than what is on the surface. A killer may look like a gigantic monster on the surface and actually be a frightened child, desperate for connection. Imagine what would happen if we all felt the threat of climate crisis in this way and allowed our sensation to guide us to solutions. We would be out of crisis very quickly if we did this as a global, unified community. I am certain of this and have tried to create a foundation for this possibility in an organization called Climate Change and Consciousness, which was mentioned earlier in this book.

DIFFERENTIATION

The movement from the purity of the undifferentiated state to the clarity of the differentiated state is a dance. Each stage of differentiation requires focus. The challenge of differentiation is the challenge of identifying distractions and choosing to focus. Without focus there is no differentiation. Differentiation is the victory of embodiment. Ironically embodied differentiation is the route to reclaiming the purity of the undifferentiated state. It is in the clarity of differentiation that you reclaim undifferentiated consciousness in an embodied state.

STEPHANIE MINES

Embryogenesis itself is a constant process of differentiation. Embryos fuel continuous specialization from within themselves as a natural function of their growth, even developing unique adaptations to novel environmental conditions. Differentiation continues throughout life in response to a variety of factors, including genetics and epigenetics. By extension, differentiation is an ongoing specialization. It is a model for how we identify ourselves and discern who we are, distinguishing ourselves from others and from the circumstances around us. In psychology this has given rise to theories of individuation and boundary setting, dependence, and codependence. These are linked to concepts, theories, and ongoing research about attachment and bonding in developing selfhood.

In regard to the secret of resilience and embryonic, Original Brilliance, I reference differentiation as the capacity to extract entelechy, or purpose-driven expression of being. Entelechy is an innate, vital life force that propels itself constantly toward self-fulfillment. It is not a static concept, and neither is differentiation.

In combination with the presence and focus of sensory acuity, differentiation leads to resilience because alignment with entelechy imparts the buoyancy inherent in purpose. This is what allows people to survive and thrive after suffering crushing shock and trauma and experience even greater vitality than they had before. Refugia, Cora, and Paul, for instance, are models of this alchemical process of ongoing differentiation that leads to claiming entelechy.

VOICING TRUTH:
ARTICULATING ORIGINAL BRILLIANCE

You have the power to stop intergenerational trauma and historical trauma in its tracks, and to keep it from spreading from your body into others. Above all, you have the power to heal. But first you have to choose to heal.

RESMAA MENAKEM

Resilience is an active principle. It is alive, multifaceted, and, most of all, it is expressive. Voicing truth, in whatever way matches entelechy, is central to the secret of resilience. In every story told here—and most definitely in my personal story in the memoir aspect of this book—when truth is voiced, resilience is accelerated by an order of magnitude. And that order of magnitude is increased incrementally and exponentially each time truth is voiced. That truth, as you will see in the final entry here on Ongoing Emergence, is not static; it evolves with every differentiation in ongoing embryogenesis, fueled by the magnificence and limitlessness of your original brilliance.

KINSHIP WITH THE NATURAL WORLD

We've created a cultural and economic landscape that is hospitable to the growth of neither leeks nor honor. If the earth is nothing more than inanimate matter, if lives are nothing more than commodities, then the way of the Honorable Harvest, too, is dead. But when you stand in the stirring spring woods, you know otherwise.

ROBIN WALL KIMMERER

It is an animate earth that we hear calling to us to feed the martens and kiss the rice. Wild leeks and wild ideas are in jeopardy. We have to transplant them both and nurture their return to the lands of their birth. We have to carry them across the wall, restoring the Honorable Harvest, bringing back the medicine.

ROBIN WALL KIMMERER

True entelechy and Embryonic Intelligence are in loving familial bonds with the natural world. It is from this enduring and innate kinship that we resurrect ourselves from the ravages of what ignorance has created. This was my discovery, as well as Paul's and Natasha's. It is spelled out in the TARA Approach, which describes in such exquisite detail how the elements are alive within us. This is inborn and enduring resilience, that same incredible buoyancy we see all around us if we open our eyes.

When I received the original guidance to create Climate Change and Consciousness, an international community of visionary activists, this was one of the principles: that each person must find their own kinship with the natural world. The veils will thin, part, and then disappear when this happens for you.

ONGOING EMERGENCE

The ability of nerve cells to change the strength and even the number of synapses is the mechanism underlying growth and learning.

ERIC KANDEL

A great genius like Wolfgang Amadeus Mozart is not who he is because of genes, but because he practiced the skills for which he became famous frequently enough to make his brain pliable and responsive.

ERIC KANDEL

Embryogenesis is ongoing; when we are directed by Embryonic Intelligence, resilience is an unending phenomenon. This transcends the recent discoveries about neuroplasticity. This is about limitless creativity and innovation. It is about the resilience of pure presence, focused sensory acuity, and continuous differentiation. It is the art of being an embryo. It is the way we can meet climate crisis and fulfill our bond, commitment, and function as voices for our living Earth.

If everyone who truly gets that we are living at a pivotal moment found their place in the movement, amazing things would happen.

REBECCA SOLNIT

The Great Turning

I watch the sea
Until the sharp winds cut my eyes to tears.
Will we be swallowed, self-cursed by privilege?
Desperate consumers so greedy for
Belonging that we
Like Ophelia
Are drowned in our sorrow?
But the sea forgives us
And retreats
Knowing our souls are
Precious umbrellas
Ready to open in this
Downpour of the Great Turning.

STEPHANIE MINES

The Perspective of an Indigenous Taoist

By Spring Cheng, Ph.D.

O n a crisp day in early March 2019, I met Stephanie Mines in a
Pacific Northwest town called Bellingham. Stephanie recruited
me as a presenter at the Climate Change and Consciousness conference,
an international gathering taking place in Findhorn, Scotland. A month
later, four hundred people from forty-some countries and more than a
dozen professional fields attended. Stephanie was the vision holder and
the main organizer of that conference.

While I was sitting in the car and chatting with this woman who is
my mother's age, I felt a surge of youthful energy, a childlike liveliness,
and an unbreakable fortitude, all integrated into a bright light emanating from Stephanie.

The meeting with Stephanie coincided with a significant turning
point in my life. At that time, I had just published my first book, *The
Resonance Code: Empowering Leaders to Evolve Toward Wholeness.*
This book was about to catapult me into a new career in which I
could reimagine the wisdom of the ancient Taoist tradition, with an
emphasis on the feminine perspective. I saw the potential benefit of

this perspective in the field of coaching, leadership, and organizational development.

I was born in China and immigrated to the United States at age twenty-two. In my first career, I had been a scientist doing biomedical research for the pharmaceutical industry. In my second career, I swung 180 degrees and became an acupuncturist and Chinese medicine doctor, retracing the footsteps of both of my maternal and paternal grandfathers, who practiced traditional medicine in China.

Through these two careers, I witnessed and experienced the painful inequality between mainstream and holistic medicine. As a holistic medicine practitioner, I contributed equally, if not more, to people's well-being and health than the mainstream medical industry. Yet the financial return and social recognition was a thin slice of what I earned working at the pharmaceutical company.

This injustice cut deep into my heart and enraged me. I felt the grief of my grandfathers. Moreover, I was alarmed. My intuition told me a health care system that does not value holistic medicine would fail because it cannot live up to its purpose: caring for human health. Therefore, it would not be a sustainable paradigm. I anticipated that this model, focusing more on illness than on sustaining good health, would collapse under its own weight. I saw a need to reimagine a health care system that focuses on wellness and empowers us to take charge in caring for our own health and bodies.

In the holistic worldview of ancient China, society and the human body follow the same set of self-organizing principles. These principles formed the core knowledge necessary to train medical practitioners, as well as politicians and community leaders. The practice of medicine and leadership were much the same. Yet, in modern times, these practices have been disrupted. Education and training in these fields focuses student minds to become obsessed with categorization and making distinctions, without adequate integration. Professional fields have become so specialized that social science and medical science can no longer share the same language, much less hold a holistic worldview.

Following my inner guidance, I chose a path on which I seek to revive this ancient practice of holistic leadership. I wrote my book to make my mark and send out a message, a vibration that calls for something entirely new.

Writing my first book took everything I had. In my fatigue, my heart was riddled with doubt, worry, and fear. "Will the world be able to see what I was trying to present? How do I even begin to knock open the thick door of our current patriarchal structure? How can I heal my own wounding incurred through my long, lonely, and hard battle with the existing system?"

The enlivening and bright light emanating from Stephanie was the dose of medicine I needed. I didn't understand it in that first encounter. But that hardly stopped me from drinking in that medicine. I have practiced energy medicine for self-healing since I was a teenager living in China. When my body produces a strong signal, my mind listens and observes without insisting to understand why at first.

In the past three years Stephanie and I have become close friends and colleagues. We mutually nourish and enliven each other through our friendship and collaboration. We learned each other's work and ran trainings together, integrating holistic medicine and women's leadership. Gradually the ingredients behind the strong dose of medicine in Stephanie revealed themselves to me.

Stephanie and I share the same vision for the evolution of human consciousness. Even though our pathways and modalities are different, we both follow the same inextinguishable, maternal instincts that led us to trust what Stephanie called the Original Brilliance in the early stages of human life—the embryonic state of our being.

Through this long patriarchal era I believe humanity has forgotten our Original Brilliance. Severing ourselves from its memory, I believe we have become trapped in an unending nightmare of separation and division, culminating in the trauma incurred from the past several hundred years of colonization.

For me, colonization does not just point to the invasion of the indigenous lands and brutalization of indigenous people. Today, the mind-set behind colonization perpetuates itself in more invisible ways, robbing us of individual indigeneity—the Original Brilliance—disrupting wholeness within every single human being embedded in the mainstream, societal structure. No matter what race we are, humanity itself has become the victim of the colonization mind-set.

The medical paradigm I acquired in college and graduate schools does not include any consideration of Original Brilliance. Despite the most advanced degree I had, I was never taught how to awaken the healing and regenerative power innate within our bodies. Instead, when the current form of medicine assaults the biological system with heavy doses of chemical treatment, it further damages our ability to connect with Original Brilliance.

Furthermore, when many of us are chained to a lifestyle that overstimulates the senses, while living at a fast pace, engaged in excessive activity and the overconsumption of substances, we continue to block our nervous systems from accessing Original Brilliance.

Recently I attended a meeting with twenty top-notch scientists working at a state-of-the-art biomedical research facility in Europe. In a brief survey, it turned out that none of these scientists practice the five simplest habits that will help maintain wellness: not smoking, drinking less than two glasses of wine in the evening, aerobic exercise at least three times a week, eating five portions of fruit and vegetables each day, and meditating for at least twenty minutes a day. If the people our society relies on for health care do not have the resources or interest to care for their own well-being, isn't that a sign that our medical paradigm itself is diseased?

Stephanie's work marks a tremendous turning point, a point of remembering and reuniting with the regenerative power of embryonic

Original Brilliance. Stephanie herself is an embodied vessel of the very thing she talks about. Every person who ever worked with Stephanie remarks on how much vitality and fortitude she embodies and inspires in others.

Another point where my life's journey and Stephanie's converge is in the integration of Eastern traditional medicine and modern science, primarily a Western construct.

Holistic medicine itself is a living entity that continues to evolve. Its traditional form may not always sufficiently meet the needs of modern people. What I love about Stephanie's approach is that she simultaneously respects the original teachings transmitted to her while taking it to a new level through integrating those teachings with her training in neuroscience and embryology.

Stephanie's knowledge came from her embodied experience of being a mother, Wounded Healer, and practitioner of energy medicine who loves the art and whose dedicated practice brings about new insights to the field. This sets her work apart from the kind of academic work into which I was trained and indoctrinated. I feel in my bones that this is the true future of science, where objective thinking and embodied subjective personal experience become integrated. This integration may help humanity come to a fuller understanding of a more holistic and connected view of the human being as a reflection of Nature herself.

Stephanie's teaching feels like medicine to me. With this medicine, I am more open to embrace a renewed Original Brilliance. I hope the readers of Stephanie's new book will drink in Stephanie's medicine and be as nourished by it as I am!

SPRING CHENG, PH.D., is a coach and teacher in leadership development and self-awareness. She spent the first half of her life in traditional, pre-industrialized China and the latter half in the United States. After receiving a doctoral degree in molecular biology and a master's in biostatistics, she worked in the pharmaceutical industry as a data scientist. However, in her career as a scientist, her heart and spirit felt empty, and she decided to dedicate herself to reconnecting with her indigenous roots through Chinese medicine and Taoism. Later, with her partner, Joe Shirley, Spring cofounded the Resonance Path Institute, where she created a holistic blend of her diverse experiences as a dancer, artist, scientist, and Chinese medicine practitioner through coaching and leadership development.

Spring invented the Resonance Code, a rebirth of the ancient Chinese classic I Ching, the Book of Changes, in the context of leadership development and conscious evolution and authored *The Resonance Code: Empowering Leaders to Evolve Toward Wholeness*. She is an advocate for integrating indigenous wisdom with modern thinking in coaching practice. She now roots her work in her native Chinese culture while spreading her influence in the Western world. For more on her work, visit her website: **www.ResonancePath.com**.

Glossary

ACT UP: AIDS Coalition to Unleash Power (ACT UP) is an international, grassroots political group working to end the AIDS pandemic. They work to improve the lives of people with AIDS through direct action, medical research, treatment, advocacy, and working to change legislation and public policies.

AIDS: Acquired immunodeficiency syndrome (AIDS) is a chronic, potentially life-threatening condition caused by the human immunodeficiency virus (HIV). By damaging your immune system, HIV interferes with your body's ability to fight infection and disease.

AIDS Medicine and Miracles: For more than twenty years AIDS Medicine and Miracles provided life-changing empowerment programs for all people with AIDS, their family members, and service providers. Powerful experiential programs were designed to build community and provide resources for hope, health, and fulfillment. AIDS Medicine and Miracles helped to address the profound effect this pandemic had on the lives of people everywhere.

alchemy: The medieval forerunner of chemistry, based on the supposed transformation of matter. It was concerned particularly with attempts to convert base metals into gold or to find a universal elixir. In the healing context, alchemy refers to transmuting pain, trauma, and related experiences into their opposite. This is one of the formulas for the Wounded Healer identity.

allostasis: The process by which the body responds to stress so as to regain homeostasis.

allostatic load: The cost of chronic exposure to elevated or fluctuating endocrine or neural responses resulting from chronic or repeated challenges that the individual experiences as stressful.

apoptosis: The death of cells, which occurs as a normal and controlled part of an organism's growth or development.

attachment: The emotional bond between a human infant or a young nonhuman animal and its parent figure or caregiver. It is developed as a step in establishing a feeling of security and demonstrated by calmness while in the parent's or caregiver's presence. Attachment also denotes the tendency to form such bonds with certain other individuals in infancy, as well as the tendency in adulthood to seek emotionally supportive social relationships.

autoimmune: Relating to disease caused by antibodies or lymphocytes produced against substances naturally present in the body. In autoimmune conditions the immune system sabotages itself, rather than being protective.

bonding: The process in which attachments or other close relationships are formed between individuals, especially between mother and infant. An early, positive relationship between a mother and a newborn child is considered by some theorists to be essential in establishing unconditional love on the part of the parent, as well as security and trust on the part of the child. In subsequent development, bonding establishes friendship and trust.

caudal: Pertaining to a tail; situated at or toward the tail end of an organism.

climate crisis: A situation characterized by the threat of highly dangerous, irreversible changes to the global climate.

consciousness: (a) The state of being awake and aware of one's surroundings. (b) The awareness or perception of something by a person. (c) The fact of awareness by the mind of itself and the world.

corona radiata: The corona radiata is the innermost layer of the cells of the cumulus oophorus and is directly adjacent to the zona pellucida, the inner protective glycoprotein layer of the ovum. Cumulus oophorus are the cells surrounding corona radiata and are the cells between corona radiata and follicular antrum.

cranial nerves: Each of twelve pairs of nerves, which arise directly from the brain, not from the spinal cord, and pass through separate apertures in the skull.

discovery: Discovery is the term that references the moment when a pregnant woman discovers she is with child. It is interesting to look at this word in the context of research. There it refers to an early phase in research settings where a new or different way of thinking (beliefs, information, knowledge) about a subject of study or research is introduced. Similarly, the moment of discovery in pregnancy is the awareness that something completely new has been found, discovered, or revealed.

dorsal: Denoting the hind region or the back surface of the body. In reference to the latter, this term sometimes is used interchangeably with posterior.

ecosystem: A biological community of interacting organisms and their physical environment.

ectoderm: The outermost layer of cells or tissue of an embryo in early development, or the parts derived from this, which include the epidermis and nerve tissue.

embryo: The prenatal being that evolves as a result of the pre-embryonic period in the first two weeks after conception. This is a time of cell maturation and differentiation, which is embryogenesis. Embryos fuel growth and differentiation at amazingly rapid rates. The embryo is the architect of the proliferation of being. After the eighth week of development the term that is generally used for the developing being is *fetus,* but in fact embryonic, or growth-oriented, development abounds throughout prenatal life.

embryogenesis: The formation and development of an embryo.

embryologist: A scientist who studies the development of animals, including humans, between the fertilization of the egg and the time when the being is born.

endocytosis: The taking in of matter by a living cell by invagination of its membrane to form a vacuole.

endoderm: The innermost layer of cells or tissue of an embryo in early development, or the parts derived from this, which include the lining of the gut and associated structures.

entelechy: (a) The realization of potential. (b) The vital principle that guides the development and functioning of an organism or other system or organization. (c) The soul.

epigenetics: The study of changes in organisms caused by modification of gene expression rather than alteration of the genetic code itself.

exposome: The measure of all the exposures of an individual in a lifetime and how those exposures relate to health. An individual's exposure begins before birth and includes insults from environmental and occupational sources. Understanding how exposures from our environment, diet, and lifestyle—among other factors—interact with our own unique characteristics, such as genetics, physiology, and epigenetics. How this affects our health is how the exposome will be articulated.

Extraordinary Meridians: The Eight Extraordinary Meridians represent the body's deepest level of energetic structuring. These meridians are the first to form in utero and are carriers of ancestral energy, which corresponds to our genetic and epigenetic inheritance. They function as deep reservoirs from which the twelve main meridians can be replenished and into which the latter can drain their excesses. There are multiple versions of the Extraordinary Meridians, but all meet this definition.

gender fluidity: Gender fluidity refers to change over time in a person's gender expression or gender identity, or both. That change might be in expression but not identity, or in identity but not expression. Or both expression and identity might change together.

implantation: The attachment of the fertilized egg, or blastocyst, to the wall of the uterus at the start of pregnancy, or somewhat later, depending on a variety of factors.

inflammation: Inflammation is a process by which your body's white blood cells and the things they make protect you from infection from outside invaders, such as bacteria and viruses.

Interbeing: A state of connectedness and interdependence of all phenomena. A being that is interconnected with others.

mesoderm: The middle layer of an embryo in early development, between the endoderm and ectoderm.

metallurgy: The branch of science and technology concerned with the properties of metals and their production and purification. As a metaphor this refers to something akin to alchemy in the transformation of suffering.

mycorrhizal: Mycorrhizae are symbiotic relationships between fungi and plants. Fungi colonize the root systems of plants, increasing nutrients and nutrient absorption. Mycorrhizal relationships are those in which the uptake of nutrients is enhanced as a result of the relationship. Mycorrhizal relationships strengthen and protect vulnerable, threatened, or diseased plants. The metaphor translates to relationships in other spheres.

nervous system: The network of nerve cells and fibers, which transmits nerve impulses between parts of the body.

organogenesis: The production and development of the organs of an animal or plant.

oxytocin: A hormone released by the pituitary gland that causes increased contraction of the uterus during labor and stimulates the ejection of milk into the ducts of the breasts. Oxytocin is often referred to as the love hormone because of its fluidity during loving contact and connection.

placenta: An organ that develops in the uterus of the mother during pregnancy. This structure provides oxygen and nutrients to a growing baby and removes waste products from the baby's blood. The placenta attaches to the wall of the uterus, and the baby's umbilical cord arises from it.

polyvagal system: The polyvagal theory proposes that the evolution of the mammalian autonomic nervous system provides the neurophysiological substrates for adaptive behavioral strategies. It further proposes that physiological state limits the range of behavior and psychological experience.

postpartum depression: Depression suffered by a mother following childbirth, typically arising from the combination of hormonal changes, psychological adjustment to motherhood, and fatigue.

pre- and perinatal psychology: Prenatal and perinatal psychology explores the psychological and psychophysiological effects and implications of the earliest experiences of the individual, before birth (prenatal), as well as during and immediately after childbirth (perinatal).

primal period: The period of human development when the basic adaptive systems reach their maturity; it includes embryonic life, the perinatal period, and the year following birth.

psychoneuroimmunology: Psychoneuroimmunology (PNI) is a discipline that has evolved in the past forty years to study the relationship among immunity, the endocrine system, and the central and peripheral nervous systems.

regeneration: The action or process of regenerating or being regenerated, particularly the formation of new animal or plant tissue. Regeneration also refers to new thinking, new paradigms, and innovations that produce flourishing new growth.

resilience: The capacity to recover quickly from difficulties—buoyancy. The ability to bounce back from stress, trauma, or even shock.

Rolfing: A form of bodywork that reorganizes the connective tissues, called fascia, that permeate the entire body.

secondary traumatization: The indirect exposure to trauma through a firsthand account or narrative of a traumatic event. This can also occur from witnessing trauma and shock or hearing it.

self-regulation: The fact of something such as an organization regulating itself without intervention from external bodies. In psychological terms this refers to the capacity to manage your own activation by noticing it, calming it, and redirecting it in a healthy way.

shock: The body's response to cumulative, repetitive trauma or experiences that completely overwhelm the capacity of that individual's nervous system to identify resources.

social engagement system: The social engagement system is a two-way interaction system (receptive and expressive) based mainly in the eyes, ears, larynx, and mouth but incorporating the entire face and the torso above the diaphragm. The social engagement system is physiologically powered by the twelve cranial nerves.

T cells: T cell, also called T lymphocyte, which is a type of leukocyte (white blood cell) that is an essential part of the immune system. T cells are one of two primary types of lymphocytes—B cells being the second type—that determine the specificity of immune response to antigens (foreign substances) in the body.

traumatic repetition: Traumatic repetitions could be seen as the result of an attempt to retrospectively "master" the original trauma, a child's play, for instance, as an attempt to turn passivity into activity. It is also the behavioral repetition of the trauma by a person of any age, either consciously or unconsciously, as a doomed way to change the circumstances. Traumatic repetition is usually the result of neuronal consolidation or habituated patterns. Addictions are a form of traumatic repetition.

unified field of consciousness: Unified field theory is derived from physics. It is a way of describing how multiple forces and relationships are a response to one field, such as gravity or electricity. Sometimes unified field theory is called the theory of everything because it reconciles incompatible phenomena. In terms of consciousness the unified field refers to interconnectedness.

ventral: Of, on, or relating to the underside of an animal or plant—abdominal.

Wounded Healer: The Wounded Healer archetype, originally proposed by Carl Jung, refers to how the lived experience of trauma, shock, and woundedness increases one's capacity to provide healing resources for others and is possibly more valuable than other forms of education for therapy. The Wounded Healer, who examines, contemplates, and extracts wisdom from the experiences of wounding, transmutes those experiences into services for others and is often guided to offer those services as a result of the wounding.

Bibliography

Barrows, Anita, and Joanna Macy, trans. 2016. *In Praise of Mortality: Selections from Rainer Maria Rilke's Duino Elegies and Sonnets to Orpheus,* revised edition. New York: Echo Point Books and Media.

Berry, Thomas. 2015. *The Dream of the Earth.* San Francisco, Calif.: Sierra Club Books.

Blackie, Sharon. 2019. *If Women Rose Rooted: A Life-changing Journey to Authenticity and Belonging.* Tewkesbury, England: September Publishing.

Blechschmidt, Erich. 1961. *The Stages of Human Development before Birth: An Introduction to Human Embryology.* Basel, CH: Karger.

———. 1977. *The Beginnings of Human Life.* Berlin/Heidelberg, DE: Springer-Verlag.

———. 2004. *The Ontogenetic Basis of Human Anatomy: A Biodynamic Approach to Development from Conception to Birth,* edited by Brian Freeman. Murrieta, Calif.: Pacific Distributing.

———. 2020. *Studies in Biodynamic Embryology.* Munich, DE: Kiener.

Blechschmidt, Erich, and Raymond F. Gasser. 2012. *Biokinetics and Biodynamics of Human Differentiation: Principles and Applications.* Berkeley, Calif.: North Atlantic books.

Burmeister, Mary Iino. 1977–2000. "Personal Collection of Mary Iino Burmeister Lecture Notes," collected by Stephanie Mines, Ph.D., The TARA Approach for the Resolution of Shock and Trauma, Gresham, Ore.

Cecchi, Lorenzo, Gennaro D'Amato, and Isabella Annesi-Maesano, 2018. "External Exposome and Allergic Respiratory and Skin Diseases." *Journal of Allergy and Clinical Immunology* 14 (3): 846–57.

Farrell, Yvonne R. 2016. *Psycho-Emotional Pain and the Eight Extraordinary Vessels,* 1st ed. London and Philadelphia: Singing Dragon.

Ghosh, Amitav. 2017. *The Great Derangement: Climate Change and the Unthinkable*. Chicago: The University of Chicago Press.

Gillespie, Sally. 2020. *Climate Crisis and Consciousness: Re-imagining Our World and Ourselves*. Oxfordshire: Routledge.

Grossinger, Richard. 2000. *Embryogenesis: Species, Gender, and Identity*. Berkeley, Calif.: North Atlantic Books.

Harjo, Joy. 1990. *In Mad Love and War*. Hanover, N.H.: University Press of New England.

———. 1994. *The Woman Who Fell from the Sky: Poems*. New York: W. W. Norton and Company.

———. 2001. *A Map to the Next World: Poetry and Tales*. New York: W. W. Norton and Company.

———. 2004. *How We Became Human: New and Selected Poems*. New York: W. W. Norton and Company.

———. 2008. *She Had Some Horses*. New York: W. W. Norton and Company.

———. 2013. *Crazy Brave: A Memoir*. New York: W. W. Norton and Company.

———. 2013. *Soul Talk, Song Language: Conversations with Joy Harjo*. Middletown, Conn.: Wesleyan University Press.

———. 2017. *Conflict Resolution for Holy Beings: Poems*. New York: W. W. Norton and Company.

———. 2019. *An American Sunrise: Poems*. New York: W. W. Norton and Company.

———. 2021. *Poet Warrior: A Memoir*. New York: W. W. Norton and Company.

———, ed. 2021. *Living Nations, Living Words: An Anthology of First People's Poetry*. New York: W. W. Norton and Company.

Hedin, Clare. 2021–2022. "Personal Communication between Clare Hedin and Stephanie Mines Ph.D."

Kandel, Eric R. 2007. *In Search of Memory: The Emergence of a New Science of Mind*. Illustrated ed. New York: W. W. Norton and Company.

Karr-Morse, Robin, and Meredith S. Wiley. 2013. *Ghosts from the Nursery: Tracing the Roots of Violence*. Revised and Updated ed. New York: Atlantic Monthly Press.

Kimmerer, Robin Wall. 2013. *Braiding Sweetgrass: Indigenous Wisdom, Scientific Knowledge and the Teachings of Plants*. Minneapolis: Milkweed Editions.

Larsen, William J. 2001. *Human Embryology*, 3rd ed. London: Churchill Livingstone.

Macy, Joanna. 1983. *Despair and Personal Power in the Nuclear Age*. First edition. Gabriola Island, BC: New Society Pub.

———. 1991. *Mutual Causality in Buddhism and General Systems Theory: The*

Dharma of Natural Systems (Suny Series, Buddhist Studies) (SUNY Series in Buddhist Studies). First edition. Albany: State University of New York Press.

———. 2007. *Widening Circles: A Memoir*. Gabriola Island, BC: New Catalyst Books.

———. 2013. *Greening of the Self*. Berkeley: Parallax Press.

———. 2021. *A Wild Love for the World: Joanna Macy and the Work of Our Time*. Edited by Stephanie Kaza. Boulder: Shambhala.

———. 2021. *World as Lover, World as Self: 30th Anniversary Edition: Courage for Global Justice and Planetary Renewal*. Edited by Stephanie Kanza. Berkeley: Parallax Press.

———. 2022. *World as Lover, World as Self: Courage for Global Justice and Ecological Renewal by Macy, Joannal Paperback*. Revised edition. Berkeley: Parallax Press.

Macy, Joanna, and Chris Johnstone. 2012. *Active Hope: How to Face the Mess We're in without Going Crazy*. Novato, Calif.: New World Library.

Macy, Joanna, and Molly Young Brown. 1998. *Coming Back to Life: Practices to Reconnect Our Lives, Our World*. First paperback edition. Gabriola Island, BC: New Society Publishers.

———. 2014. *Coming Back to Life: The Updated Guide to the Work That Reconnects,* Revised edition. Gabriola Island, BC: New Society Publishers.

Macy, Joanna, and Norbert Gahbler. 2006. *Pass it On: Five Stories That Can Change the World*. Berkeley: Parallax Press.

Madaule, Paul. 2015. *When Listening Comes Alive*. Minneapolis: Publish Green.

Marya, Rupa, and Raj Patel. 2021. *Inflamed: Deep Medicine and the Anatomy of Injustice*. New York: Farrar, Straus, and Giroux.

Maté, Gabor. 2018. *In the Realm of Hungry Ghosts: Close Encounters with Addiction*. New York: Vintage Canada.

———. 2019. *When the Body Says No: The Cost of Hidden Stress*. London: Vermilion.

Maté, Gabor, and Daniel Maté. 2023. *The Myth of Normal: Trauma, Illness, and Healing in a Toxic Culture*. New York: Vintage Canada.

Menzam-Sills, Cherionna. 2021. *Spirit Into Form*. Independently Published.

Mines, Stephanie. 1996. *Sexual Abuse/Sacred Wound: Transforming Deep Trauma*. Barrytown, N.Y.: Station Hill Press.

———. 2006. *TARA Approach Training Manual: Pre- and Perinatal Psychology*. TARA Approach.

———. 2010. *TARA Approach Training Manual: The Miracle of Birth*. TARA Approach.

———. 2014. *New Frontiers in Sensory Integration: Limbic Stimulation, Authentic Relationship, and a Multi-Disciplinary Treatment Design*. Stillwater, Okla.: New Forums Press.

———. 2015. *They Were Families: How War Comes Home*. Stillwater, Okla.: New Forums Press.

———. 2021. *We Are All in Shock: Energy Healing for Traumatic Times*. Cedar Rapids: New Page Books.

Moore, Keith. L. 2019. *The Developing Human: Clinically Oriented Embryology*. Philadelphia: W. B. Saunders Company.

Moore, Keith. L., T. V. N. Persaud, and Mark Torchia. 2020. *Before We Are Born: Essentials of Embryology and Birth Defects*. Amsterdam: Elsevier.

Nugent, Nicole R., Jennifer A. Sumner, and Ananda B. Amstadter. 2014. "Resilience After Trauma: From Surviving to Thriving." *European Journal of Psychotraumatology* 5 (1): 25, 339.

Seed, John, Joanna Macy, Pat Fleming, and Anne Naess. 2007. *Thinking Like a Mountain: Towards a Council of All Beings*. Gabriola Island, BC: New Catalyst Books.

Senier, Laura, Phil Brown, Sara Shostak, and Bridget Hanna. 2016. "The Socio-Exposome: Advancing Exposure Science and Environmental Justice in a Postgenomic Era." *Environmental Sociology* 3 (2): 107–21.

Shiva, Vandana. 2016. *Soil Not Oil*. Berkeley: North Atlantic Books.

Soh, Kwang-Sup. 2004. "Bonghan Duct and Acupuncture Meridian as Optical Channel of Biophoton." *Journal of the Korean Physical Society* 45 (5): 1196–98.

Thunberg, Greta. 2019. *No One Is Too Small to Make a Difference*. New York: Penguin Books.

Tomatis, A. Alfred. 1991. *The Conscious Ear: My Life of Transformation through Listening*. Barrytown, N.Y.: Station Hill Press.

———. 1996. *The Ear and Language*. Moulin Publishing.

———. 2005. *The Ear and the Voice*. Translated by Roberta Prada, Pierre Sollier, and Francis Keeping. Lanham, Md.: Scarecrow Press.

Van der Wal, Jaap. 2021–2022. "Personal Collection of Jaap van der Wal Lecture Notes." Collected by Stephanie Mines, Ph.D., The TARA Approach for the Resolution of Shock and Trauma, Gresham, Ore..

Weinstein, Anne Diamond. 2016. *Prenatal Development and Parents' Lived Experiences: How Early Events Shape our Psychophysiology and Relationships*. New York: W. W. Norton and Company.

Yehuda, Rachel, and Amy Lehrner. 2018. "Intergenerational Transmission of Trauma Effects: Putative Role of Epigenetic Mechanisms." *World Psychiatry* 17 (3): 243–57.

Index

Page numbers in *italics* refer to illustrations.

OTHER BOOKS BY STEPHANIE MINES

Sexual Abuse/Sacred Wound: Transforming Deep Trauma

We Are All in Shock: Energy Healing for Traumatic Times

New Frontiers in Sensory Integration

They Were Families: How War Comes Home

*The Dreaming Child: How Children Can Help Themselves
Recover from Illness and Injury*

Two Births by Janet Brown, Eugene Lesser, and Stephanie Mines